PRAISES

"Sharon's speech got me charged up. It [...] back in life in accomplishing anything is yourself. It was very motivating." *Atlanta / Women of Empowerment Luncheon*

"Over 75% of the evaluations from our Empowerment Luncheon mentioned Sharon Frame as the speaker that affected them in an impactful, life changing, and positive manner."

"Her charismatic manner and quick wit captured our audience. She has the natural ability to share wisdom and insight, while inspiring and empowering your spirit." *Lynda Shorter CEO, Voices Of Influence Speakers Bureau*

"Sharon has this way of reaching into your soul, grabbing the tiniest light of potential, and making it shine before your eyes, giving you a brand new perspective that your dreams are actually achievable. She has helped me to change my limited thinking." *Priscilla Kamale / Money Systems/ London, England*

"Sharon is hands down one of the most exceptional and effective communicators that I know. She knows how to engage an audience and she is engaging. She knows how to compel. She knows how to tell a story, call people to action." *Kysa Daniels/ Former CNN/HLN Anchor*

"Sharon's enthusiasm is contagious!! She is a wonderful and awesome orator and facilitator. She immediately grabs your attention and engages you throughout the entire session." *Greta Kelly, Recruitment Manager / Spelman College*

"Sharon Frame was the most outstanding speaker we've ever had here at Spelman College for our SWEPT program. She made it come alive. She was totally awesome. I would recommend her to anyone." *Tony Ireland/ Spelman College*

"Sharon is an extremely engaging speaker who enlightened our students to the possibilities of what they can do. Her dynamic and compelling delivery makes people think and challenges them to climb higher in life. She is among the best motivational speakers out there." *Dr. Jerome Greene/ Southern University Chancellor*

LEAD**HER**SHIP

OWN IT! LOVE IT! LEARN IT! GIVE IT!

Women Redefining Wealth, Health and Happiness...
And How You Can Too

Sharon Frame, Former Cnn Anchor

LeadHERship: Own It! Love It! Learn It! Give it! Women Redefining Wealth, Health and Happiness...And How You Can Too

To order additional copies of LeadHERship, or to book Sharon Frame for a dynamic keynote at your next women's conference, training session, retreat or special event, call 678 602-2899 or visit: www.sharonframe-speaks.com

ISBN: 978-0-9826780-3-9

Printed and Bound in the United States of America

Logo Design: SELF Graphic Design selfgraphics.wix.com/selfgraphics
Book Cover Design: Tracy A. Hanes of T. Allen Hanes & Associates
Interior Design: A Reader's Perspective

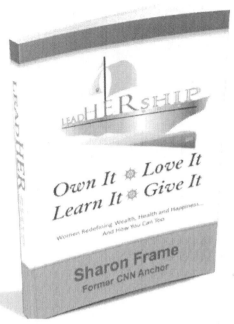

"LeadHERship is a new twist on an age old concept. This book reveals a fresh perspective on leadership from a woman's point of view. The stories from women who overcame enormous obstacles and created the lives they wanted are instructive as well as inspiring.

This book is a tremendous example of how powerful and effective women are and will serve to help women everywhere find their own LeadHERship Power. **"**
Lisa Giruzzi, Best Selling Author, Speaker and Leading Communication Authority

Redefining Life's
LeadHERship
Journey

"What is it that I want to achieve? I want to live in higher awareness and be connected to my Source; live in the space as a way of living and being in the world.

Why? So that I get to know who I truly am for myself and others. So that I am not constantly running against the current of life and feel battered, tired and depleted; So that I have real peace and joy in my life.

Once I have that as a natural flow, I can then truly be the contribution I am for others and create relationships that work and make a difference."

- Uma Davis/New Mexico

LEADHERSHIP

Acknowledgments

THIS BOOK "LEADHERSHIP" would not have been possible without the guiding hand of God. It is He who continues to steer my life in the right direction. It is He who challenges me to sail uncharted waters; to use the power of the pen to reassure the faithful, refresh the weary and rescue those stranded at sea.

To the ladies featured in this book who candidly shared their back stories of struggle to triumph, you are a beacon of light. Lives will be changed because you took the trouble to find your true north.

To my many sisters whose bonds of friendships create the waves that lift me higher, I am forever grateful.

To the women whose love and stewardship charted the course before me, I am forever in your debt: My mother, Veleta Jackson, my auntie Sky Gordon and my sister Trisha Walden who embody the spirit of LeadHERship.

And to my five nieces, Laree, Monique, Amanda, Diamond and Alexis; all anchored in a rich tradition of Ownership, Relationship, Scholarship and Stewardship. "Keep the wind at your back and the sun on your face." And lead your ship as far as your unbridled spirit will take you.

Author's Note

THE JOURNEY TO pen this book started as a personal challenge. I dared myself to write a book in thirty days, in time for an upcoming speaking event. I wanted company. So I created the 30-Day Challenge and asked friends, clients and perfect strangers to join me for the ride!

The challenge runs on a system that turbo-charges your efforts and provides a daily community platform for accountability and support. It was an amazing thrill for everyone to laser-focus and concentrate on just one specific individual goal! Now the challenge is part of my on-going coaching program offered to people all over the country!

Listen to what focus partners are saying about the Focus and Follow Through 30-Day Challenge, and come join the rally to set yourself up for success...and lead your ship!

"Sharon's 30 Day Challenge helped me thrive off of the synergistic energy that was created. It's not just about the outcome; it's about the journey and how much I was able to expand my capacity while producing results. I've created the foundation and framework to reach 100 Million people with awareness of new hands-only CPR and to empower others to save more lives!"
~ Robbie MacCue, Paramedic /New York/ www.CPRMatters.org

"*My challenge was to boost my business activity to get exposure to funding opportunities. The 30-Day Challenge challenged me to push myself to prepare a polished business plan, set five year strategy and build a network and partnerships with organizations similar to mine. My success in doing so was phenomenal!*"
~ *Sheila Wilson / Norcross, Georgia /*
www.afterthestormbodyandsoul.org

My Challenge is to improve my overall health and fitness by making exercise, healthy eating and sleep a priority in my life. The power of accountability is amazing. Having a forum to post my daily focus goals and pictures of my accomplishments has helped me become more mindful of my eating habits, and has motivated me to become excited about exercising. The forum is my vision board of success. As Sharon so eloquently stated, "I'm not just trying...I'm doing it." Thank you, Sharon!"
~ *Greta Tifre / Atlanta, Georgia*

"*The Sharon Frame 30 Day Challenge is a great experience for me. Even though I consider myself goal oriented it always helps to be part of a group to hold you accountable. Even the front runners need teammates! I was able to finish a book in 27 days, from interview to publish… and was able to complete the draft of a second book in a 12 hour laser focused session. Highly recommended for anyone looking to get things done fast! And Sharon Frame is the consummate leadership coach! Thanks!*"
~ *Tracy A. Hanes / Author, Speaker, Coach - Houston, Texas*
www.tracyahanes.com

Exciting details at: www.focusandfollowthrough.biz

Setting a Better Sail

Ownership: *Barbara Singer chased a paycheck to the top of the corporate ladder only to discover she was "propped up against the wrong building." She had the big house, high-powered job, city-club membership… but no happiness. So she quit her busy, stressful life and set a course of adventure, freedom and world travel on a shoestring budget. First she moved to Florida to become a waitress at a beach bar, hatched a plan to go island- hopping in the Caribbean and then settled in Italy where she fell in love with a winemaker! Barbara reveals how she finally took charge at the helm to "lead her ship" and live her dream life, on Page 17.*

Relationship: *Josette Redwolf toured the country with some of the biggest rock n' roll bands. Her little black book contained the names of celebrities and her famous rock star boyfriends. She was riding high on life but her love tank was empty. Her desperate search for love took her to all the wrong places. She stumbled in and out of painful, abusive relationships that almost ruined her — until true love said, enough! Find out how the birth of a miracle child reversed her self-destructive behavior and delivered what her troubled, wandering soul hankered since the day she ran away from home at age thirteen. Page 26.*

Scholarship: *Dr. Shirley Cheng could be a bitter, angry woman and few people would blame her. She's blind and has been wheelchair bound since infancy. But neither blindness nor disability dims her love of life or passion for learning. Severe arthritis prevents her from using brail. Yet she wrote three books in a year, has twenty-seven book awards and has read the Bible fourteen times in twelve different translations. So what's got her so enthusiastic about life? Read about one blind woman's big vision to help people see God more clearly. Page 44.*

Stewardship: *Shanna McFarlane found herself homeless at sixteen and begging for food on the streets in a foreign country. But pity isn't welcomed here. Her struggle to defy poverty put her on the road to wealth. By the age of thirty -one Shanna was a self-made millionaire and CEO of a real estate empire. Now she uses her "rags to riches" story to lift others as she climbs. Her "lead her ship" journey is bound to inspire you, on Page 58.*

Remarkable women redefining Wealth, Health and Happiness reveal their secrets. Learn how you too can set a better sail in life, and "lead your ship" to success with clarity, confidence and conviction.

Table of Contents

Part III: Redefining Moments

Power to Lead Her Ship!

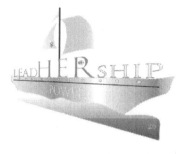

DID YOU KNOW that the highest duty of a leader is to serve? It is "service to many that leads to greatness," according to self-help guru Jim Rohn. He was quoting the greatest leader who ever served: Jesus Christ.

Do you wish to be great? Do you wish to live a life of significance? Be big enough to bow. Be willing to stoop low and serve others. That's the gauge of your greatness; a sign of a life well lived.

Greatness went searching for Mother Theresa while she was busy "being." She found a way to serve "the least among us," and her humble acts of kindness made her great. It also made her one of the most admired leaders in the 20th/21st century.

As the great Zig Ziglar famously said, "You can have everything in life you want if you will just help other people get what they want."

But before you kneel to serve others serve yourself. If your jug of kindness is half-empty or depleted you have little or nothing to pour into my cup.

So leadership really begins with serving yourself. "Physician heal thyself." Make sure you are well so you can more effectively heal others.

Women have a difficult time reconciling this truth. It's no great secret that women are nurturers by nature. "The better half" seems hard-wired to take care of everybody. Quality time is dedicated to serving husbands, children, bosses, employees, neighbors, and friends. And at the end of the day you are drained and exhausted with little love left for you.

SACRED SELFISHNESS

How many mothers, wives or female friends do you know who practice "sacred selfishness"? I'll venture to say very few. That phrase was coined by a friend from Las Vegas. It describes the "me time" she insists on seizing now and then. Sacred selfishness gives her control. It helps her become a better leader of her own life with less stress and more value.

What if you saw leadership as your responsibility to take charge of your life and determine your destiny on your terms? Forget about chasing a paycheck or running in the rat race to pursue the "American Dream."

What if you followed your heart? What if you embraced that career you know is your calling? Imagine how your service could help light the dark path for others to see more clearly and shine more brilliantly. That is LeadHERship Power!

LeadHERship is the ability to claim your space on the planet and use it to serve others.

This LeadHERship philosophy of mine is anchored on four divine principles: to OWN, to LOVE, to LEARN and to GIVE.

Get ready to meet women just like you who have tapped into their LeadHERship Power and redefined wealth, health, and happiness. They now lead lives of significance with purpose and conviction.

Some of these women faced tremendous tragedies, wrenching set-backs and frequent frustrations on their life-journeys. But they chose not to curse the stormy winds. Instead they re-charted their course and set a better sail. You have the LeadHERship Power to do the same.

The Four Anchors of LeadHERship

⚓ **own-er-SHIP** [oh-ner-ship]
(To Own) The ability to own or control your life, to take full responsibility for your past, present and future.

⚓ **re-la-tion-SHIP** [ri-ley-shuh n-ship]
(To Love) The ability to effectively relate to others through love based on self-value; the personal measure of your worth defined through your bond or connection with the Divine spirit of love, God, the Creator.

⚓ **schol-ar-SHIP** [skol-er-ship]
(To Learn) The pursuit of lifetime learning; the hunger to improve skill sets, gain new knowledge, wisdom and understanding; to embrace personal development and self-improvement.

⚓ **stew-ard-SHIP** [stoo-erd-ship, styoo-]
(To Give) The willingness to give back; to lift others as you climb; to grow, protect and use your gifts and talent to uplift humanity; to live a life of gratitude and generosity.

PART I
LEAD HER SHIP

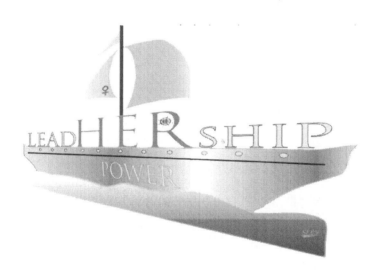

Ownership

"I find the great thing in this world is not so much where we stand, as in what direction we are moving. We must sail sometimes with the wind and sometimes against it—but we must sail, and not drift, nor lie at anchor."

~ Oliver Wendell Holmes

LIFE IS LIKE a voyage on the high seas. You chart a course and set your destination. Sometimes you drift off course. You wish for blue skies and smooth sailing. But along with the sunshine "there's gonna be a little rain sometimes." Other times dark clouds and threatening storms will roll in.

The wind of change might blow trouble your way: illness, bankruptcy, divorce, financial set-back. It's easy to blame the weather. But what matters in life is not how hard the wind blows. It's how well you respond and course-correct.

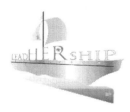

Know this, life is "opportunity mixed with difficulty."

If you ever get fed up with the difficulty, you have the opportunity to change things. But every new opportunity comes with its own set of difficulties. Here is the sweet irony: difficulty may cause set-backs, but it also offers great opportunity for growth. It opens the door to lessons that can lead to a fuller, richer life. But you must choose to take control and "lead your ship." Why live life drifting aimlessly at sea? You have the power to take the helm and steer in an entirely different direction.

That's what Barbara Singer did. She got sick and tired of her "successful" but empty, meaningless existence. So, she reinvented her life!

Life has no remote. Get up and change it yourself!"
~ Kamari aka Lyrikal

GO WHERE THE WIND BLOWS

BY BARBARA SINGER

AT FORTY FOUR years old I quit my life or I should say life quit me. On the outside I had it all: big house, big career in commission sales and a treasured teenage daughter in private school.

I appeared to be living the American dream. But while sitting at the top of the ladder, I realized that I was propped up against the wrong building.

I felt trapped, stuck on the relentless treadmill of the pursuit of success, all the while dreaming of a life of adventure, travel and freedom. In the throes of this emotional conflict, I met someone new and made the difficult and life-altering decision to [end my fractured marriage and] abandon my "comfortable" life.

Just one month after my only child went off to college the new love of my life suddenly died of a heart attack. I was in a state of shock, total upheaval and mid-life awakening. I embarked on a spiritual journey to figure out what to do with the "second half" of my life. I liquidated my home, rented it and reduced all my monthly living expenses to 3 bills: cell, health insurance and a small storage unit.

CHARTING UNKNOWN WATERS

First, I took a road trip from Pennsylvania to Alaska and back with my seventy- year-old dad. Then I moved to south Florida with visions of working at a Tiki Bar on the beach. Instead, I ended up waiting tables at a marina bar where I met Captain Pete who was living on his 42-foot Hunter sailboat. One night we hatched a plan to go island hopping in the Caribbean for 100 days in one direction.

New Year's Eve we set sail even though we barely knew each other and I had never sailed before. It wasn't all butterflies and sunshine, but I had the time of my life and would do it again in a New York minute!

Next I rented a room from a woman I found on the internet in Tuscany, Italy. I didn't speak the language or know anyone there. But it was the place I had always dreamed of living. Just ten days after my arrival, I went to a little family winery, met Giuseppe, a young, handsome third generation winemaker, fell in love and spent the rest of the summer riding the hills of Chianti on a Vespa.

Now I still have just two suitcases and a computer. And I live at the winery and use my "American Marketing Brain" to promote our wines using the internet and showcasing all the unique things that make Italians and their passion for wonderful food and wine so special.

ROWING MY OWN BOAT

I turned my journal into a published book, became a certified life reinvention coach after readers started to ask me to help them make the transition and do speaking engagements. My latest adventure is hosting a "Life Reinvention Retreat" at a one thousand-year-old monastery to share my knowledge and this magical place I call home.

I never dreamed that in such a short period of time my whole life could change. Some people say it takes courage to do what I did.

To recap, the worst thing that could ever happen happened to me: I had fallen head over heels in love with a man while I was married and turned my world upside down to be with him. It shocked everyone who knew me and wreaked havoc on my relationship with my only child who blamed me for wrecking our family. Then my new fiancé died of a sudden heart attack.

DRAMA LEFT BEHIND IN MY WAKE

With all that behind me I went about living life with a whole different perspective.

Ironically, it was also the best thing that happened to me because it lit a fire under my chair: I realized that life can change on a dime and it can be "game over" in a second and we don't get to choose the day. And if I have a goal or a dream I had better move on it yesterday.

Had I not decided to toss out society's rule book, I would still be working a job I didn't like in order to earn money, commuting and stressing about my weekly sales quota, saving money for retirement and waiting for retirement day to begin living. My soul would have died a long, slow death. I would have self-medicated with food, wine, exercise, entertainment, consumerism, Prozac or whatever distraction came into fashion.

I now collect experiences, not stuff. By no longer maintaining a traditional home and lifestyle, I live when and where I want all over the world for less than most people pay in property taxes and insurance.

I never dreamed that my life could be so full, exciting and filled with joy. As I follow my heart and co-create with the divine power, the red carpet rolls out for me and life becomes easy and fun.

BARBARA REDEFINES WEALTH, HEALTH AND HAPPINESS

As for wealth, I am no longer running on the money wheel and know that true wealth comes from time, freedom and choices.

Now I choose to give back by teaching others to live without reservations and not by society's rule book.

Teaching and inspiring others to live their best life brings me great joy because I can use my life experiences, the good, the bad and the ugly, to help others overcome fear and live the life of their dreams. Since I lived through some major transitions, I have firsthand insight and compassion.

I have taken ownership of my life. I am no longer a slave to my ego. Running on the business hamster wheel was a trick of the ego. It made me feel important. I was very busy doing all these things, but not actually productive, just active. And happiness was nowhere in sight. I am so glad I took control and changed course. Now I am really living!

BARBARA'S TEN OWNERSHIP TIPS

Taking Control at the Helm

- Take 100% responsibility for your life. You created it with your choices and you can change by choosing again.
- Evaluate the success of a day by joyfulness not productiveness.
- Be acutely aware of how you spend your precious time.
- Live with urgency, purpose and joy.
- Be totally honest with yourself. Take action and let the chips fall where they may. When you change, others must change.
- Don't live to please others. It's a dead end street.
- Change comes by choice or by force. It is what you do with it that counts.
- One door closes so another can open. The key is not to get stuck in the hallway.
- See everything that happens as a stepping-stone to the next great thing. It is all about the journey.
- Contribute to making the world a wonderful place by shining your light and being happy.

Barbara Elaine Singer is an award-winning author of Living Without Reservations. She specializes in overcoming fear, the power of affirmations and teaches others how to jump off the treadmill of consumerism and create a life of purpose and passion. www.HowToQuitYourLife.com

My Redefining Moment

Setting a Better Sail

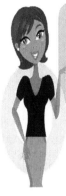

"Business is a trick of the ego. It makes you feel important. You are very busy, you are doing all these things, but you are not actually productive. You are just active."

Barbara Singer

Have you taken ownership of your life? Or are you a slave to your ego? Make a list of how you could be active but not productive.

_____

_____

_____

_____

_____

_____

_____

_____

Relationship

"I can only love you most when I love me best"
~ Steve Maraboli

LOVE IS THE most powerful force on the planet.

It is the divine spirit that links us as human beings. You can feel love in the carefree embrace of a giddy, innocent child. A lonely, elderly woman is warmed by love when a caring neighbor checks in on her now and then. Natural disasters strike a world away, and love moves us to tears. It also nudges us to open our wallets, to give to perfect strangers and help relieve their pain.

Love causes us to be patient and kind to each other. We overlook faults; extend mercy to the guilty because of love.

Love is like a warm blanket that gently snuggles us from life's cold insecurities. It gives us a feeling of belonging. Love is as necessary as the air we breathe. Go long enough without it and you will surly die.

Love is reflected in the relationships we build. It's the cement that seals and strengthens the bonds of fellowship.

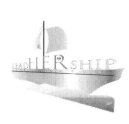

But sometimes relationships crack, crumble and go dreadfully wrong. The high rate of domestic violence in this country bears that out. Every day countless victims young and old are swept up in sorrow or left drowning in abuse.

This is NOT love.

"Love shouldn't hurt, drag you through an emotional roller coaster or leave you feeling like less of a person."

~ *Michelle Hall*

JOSETTE REDWOLF COULD write the book on broken relationships. She is a former model and artist who was on the road with some of the biggest rock n' roll stars in the music industry. Now she owns a rapidly-growing jewelry and fashion design business. Her bold and edgy pieces of semi-precious stones can be seen on Hollywood stars like Johnny Depp and Roseanne Barr. But for years her troubled life was a fractured diamond in the rough.

Josette said she was physically and mentally abused as a child and ran away from home at the age of thirteen. But she quickly became a magnet for self-destructive relationships. She stumbled in and out of them for years, desperately seeking to love and be loved. This need to belong drove her into the arms of men who used and abused her. She blindly opened her heart to the very thing she ran from as a child.

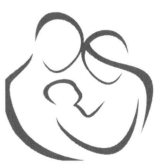

One reason why Josette craved love from others is because she had little to none for herself. So she got trapped in a vicious cycle of abuse. Repeatedly she vowed "never again" to get ensnared in another toxic relationship only to find herself right back in the same spot with a different man.

It took years of self-destruction and a debilitating illness before Josette realized her worth and learned to love herself. One pivotal moment came with the birth of her son. The innocent, authentic and unconditional love from a child changed everything. Josette finally understood a critical life-lesson: we teach people how to treat us. Sometimes we give them permission to use and abuse us. We can also give ourselves permission to accept no more of that abuse.

Josette's lesson on love and relationship had reached a new level. Her miracle child helped her understand divine love and paved the way for her to love herself even more.

THIRSTY FOR LOVE
BY JOSETTTE REDWOLF

> *"The quality of your life is the quality of your relationships."*
>
> ~*Anthony Robbins*

My name is Josette Redwolf and I love the woman I am turning out to be. I say turning out to be because at forty-seven I am reinventing myself yet again.

I was born to a runway *Playboy* model and had a very eventful life right from the very beginning. I was nearly delivered in a service elevator at Memorial Hall in Dayton, Ohio, during an Elvis Presley concert in February 1966 when my mother was dating JD Sumner of the *Stamps*.

My early life was watching my mother on the Mike Douglas Show modeling for Bettie Rogue as she wore incredible leather capes and furs and looked like a super model. She wasn't able to show affection and began to lose interest in me when I was around the age of nine. That's when she became pregnant with my sister.

That's also when the mental and physical abuse started. There are many years that are a blur. I think it's a coping mechanism to give myself a way to heal.

Living in an unhealthy relationship with someone who talked down to you all day made me want to escape just for my own sanity. There were so many times I thought about taking my own life.

LOOKING FOR LOVE

I knew I had to leave if I was to survive. So at thirteen years old I ran away from home and went on the road with rock n' roll bands. A southern rocker, who will remain nameless, took me under his wing. We were together for five wild years. At thirteen you can't really know what love is.

I worked for different rock bands as a wardrobe and personal assistant, creating clothing and jewelry accessories for some of the biggest names. I traveled on the road with bands like *Krokus*, *Quiet Riot*, *Armoured Saint*, and *Van Halen*. I even dated a few of the rockers including David Lee and Eric Carr from *Kiss*. He was another love of my life who was yet another wounded soul.

I had an incredible life on the road traveling. I later realized it wasn't that I loved being with the performers. I wanted to find out what made them tick, because I was trying to figure out why my father could abandon me as a child.

My father sang with the *Oak Ridge Boys* when they sang gospel for a short time. I had always been told he left to become a famous musician. He would send me signed records from the road of other musicians he worked with. Then one day there was nothing. He never wrote to me again.

My life took me into modeling and later I owned an all-male dance revue that did extremely well.

But I was still so much a child trying to make my way in life as an adult. I fell victim to a roommate who tried to sell me into a human trafficking ring. I got sick once with severe ovarian cysts and endometriosis. Doctors had to take out one ovary and left only a third of the other. They told me I would never have children because it was medically impossible. I was heart-broken. I knew I wanted to be a mother so badly. I wanted a child to love and nurture and to teach them that despite all of my experiences, the world could be a wonderful place.

CYCLE OF PAIN

At the age of twenty-four I moved to Arizona and used my talents I had acquired on the road as a costume designer and created my own clothing line.

I sold my business after falling in love with my landlord who talked me into taking him to California to live out his dreams of being on a yacht and selling boats for a living by the water.

I had always felt because of my childhood abuse that there was something wrong with me. So I ended up over and over again in situations that were abusive and manipulative. I was attracted to that because it's what I knew.

It was in California that doctors diagnosed me with CTD, Connective Tissue Disease. I lost feeling in my legs and was unable to walk. I was stuck in a tiny boat and couldn't even get to the bathroom on my own. My former landlord turned husband said he was fed up with helping me, so he left. Eventually I got to the point where I could walk again. And I later accepted him back because I did not want to be alone.

Because I wanted a child so badly, we considered adoption. One day I went to our attorney to get the adoption papers and bring them back to the boat for him to sign. I was finally going to be a mother! I boarded the boat, walked in and he was having sex with the mother of the child we were supposed to adopt. They didn't stop. He kept thrusting and she looked at me and asked me to join them.

WAKE UP CALL

I still cry to this day at this memory. How could I have wasted so much of my life with this man? For so long I felt entirely worthless because I had tolerated this nonsense!

At that moment I had a new awakening. I wasn't this bad person who needed this abuse over and over again. I was a good person, someone who would do anything for the people I loved. For a split second I literally sat across from the two of them as they continued to have sex and said to myself, "My God, Josette, what have you done to yourself? The past abuse wasn't enough you had to continue it all of these years?"

I realized in that moment what I was doing. I was repeating my cycle of abuse. Right then I packed a duffle bag, left San Diego and hitchhiked to Los Angeles. Sadly enough though, there had to be a few more shameful wakeup calls before I would finally break the cycle.

I had very little money when I got mugged one night and lost everything except my little dog, Ari. Not long after that I found myself on the streets homeless.

LIFE ON THE STREETS

I ended up meeting little angels from then on. Not the normal kind you would think of. I met a man named Joe who taught me how and where to go for food and how to panhandle. I wasn't homeless for very long but those weeks on the L.A. streets were the most freeing times I have ever had. I witnessed true relationships. It was pure love between people showing each other how to survive, telling stories about days long past and sharing what food they had among themselves. They even helped each other find boxes to cut up to lay their heads on at night.

One day I was panhandling in front of I-Hop and a guy offered me a job as a celebrity look-alike, since I looked a lot like Audrey Hepburn. I worked for him for a few weeks and he introduced me to some of his police friends who hired me to do some undercover work. They needed someone to pretend to be an out-of-work actress and wear a wire into a business to get information. It worked out so well they made me a full-time undercover consultant working for an apartment owner trying to get rid of a drug dealer.

I was able to successfully get information that triggered a raid of the apartment above me. The gay couple who lived there had been exchanging sex with homeless boys for drugs and taping it. Police found over 300 videotapes in the apartment. They were both HIV positive, and at the end of every tape of them having sex they would look at the camera and say, "Another one bites the dust." It disgusted me so much I offered to give up my pay check to see something very bad happen to them in jail. One died two weeks later. It might have been a coincidence.

VICIOUS CYCLE

I ended up moving away after I met a comedian/actor named Chris who was another tortured soul. My cycle of attracting hurtful relationships continued. At least Chris was not abusive. But he came with his own emotional baggage, having been abused himself as a child.

I suppose all of this time I always thought my love could heal these men in my life. But I had to finally learn that healing would have to begin with me.

One beautiful morning I woke up and my breasts hurt so much it felt like I had been beaten with a baseball bat. I had also missed my period. It turned out I was pregnant.

I couldn't believe it. It was a miracle! The Universe had blessed me with what I always wanted: to be a mom, to have a beautiful child. Doctors had told me it was medically impossible to get pregnant. So I took the pregnancy as a sign from the universe that the Universe still had faith in me; that I was a good and deserving woman and that it was time to truly clean up my life!

TURNING POINT

I went home and threw away my black book and vowed my life would change. That book contained the home phone numbers of every rock band I had ever worked for, all my former boyfriends and many celebrities. I had decided that day that not one of these people in the book was good enough, nor were they people I would want around my child. I tossed it because I had to start my life fresh and clean. Chris later proposed to me, even though he was afraid he wouldn't be a good dad.

As we went on in the pregnancy I become very ill. Every time I would walk I went into labor. So I was sent home on strict bed-rest for the remainder of my pregnancy.

MIRACLE CHILD

My son, Sterling, arrived eight weeks early at six pounds, twelve ounces. He wasn't breathing well and I was not able to hold him. When the nurses allowed me to see his beautiful little face I asked why he wasn't crying and the doctor said he must be content. But I knew he was sick.

I moved Sterling to Georgia so we'd be near my father who I did not know very well. That gave us a chance for some emotional closure. Chris had planned to join us in Georgia, to personally ask my father for my hand in marriage. But the day before he was to fly in, he died of heart failure from a drug overdose.

So there I was in Georgia alone with a sick child and

so heartbroken by Chris's death I could barely move. If there was any lingering doubt that I had to get my act together this erased it. For now a loving little baby boy depended totally on me to take care of him. And his needs became priority.

Sterling got sicker and doctors could not figure out what was wrong with him. He wasn't able to hold his head up until well after he was ten months old. He would choke and turn blue and I would have to flip him upside down and clear his throat. He didn't sleep and he would cry out in pain all the time.

A MOTHER'S DETERMINATION

It was storming badly when I took Sterling to a hospital in Atlanta to see a diagnostician. After three hours of waiting, the storm knocked out the power. The receptionist shouted out that she was sorry, and that they would have to reschedule appointments for another day.

That's when I jumped up on a desk and yelled, "Excuse me, doctors and nurses, you can arrest me if you want to, but I am not leaving here until someone looks at my child and tells me what is wrong with him. So go ahead and call the police if you have to. But I'm not moving."

A doctor quickly came over and I gave him a long list of Sterling's symptoms. I told him everyone had told me I am a first-time mom, that it's all in my head and I was just imagining my child's symptoms. My son started choking right then on the spot and was admitted. The doctor ran test after test and then told me Sterling had Myasthenia

Gravis, an autoimmune disorder, and wouldn't live to see his fifth birthday.

They put him on horrible medicine with side effects that were worse than the actual symptoms and he was so miserable. He would ask me if he was dying and I would say, "No baby." I finally said enough is enough. He was two years old, and if he was going to die he was going to die a happy child and not sick from meds.

Sterling needed occupational therapy, physical therapy and speech therapy. I had to install super plush carpet at home because he was so sensitive, even his clothes would hurt him.

DEALING WITH THE PAIN

One day when I was hauling a roll of carpet from my truck I heard the loudest pops of my life coming from my neck. I had no clue that I had hurt myself.

The next morning I woke up and I could barely move. I was in horrible pain. I went to the hospital. They did an x-ray and told me I had pulled the muscles in my neck.

For months I suffered tremors in my legs and eventually lost feeling in both legs. I was in so much pain I thought I was dying.

I finally saw a specialist who did a CAT Scan that showed I had broken my neck in three places. The doctor said one wrong jolt and I could be a veggie. I needed immediate reconstructive surgery. Both Sterling and I were later diagnosed with Ehers Danlos, a degenerative tissue disease. Finally we had a diagnosis that fit.

He wasn't going to die that soon and we had a future. We were very sick but we could work with that.

The doctor said I had so much nerve damage I was a hundred percent disabled with little hope of full recovery. Despite excruciating pain I worked my butt off and slowly began to get the feeling back in my limbs. I was not about to accept not being able to run in the park with my son or to play ball with him. I went from wheelchair to walker to cane.

ROCKY SITUATIONS

My son has always loved rock collecting. Our adventurous hunts in rock mines helped him gain strength. We had built a huge collection. One day I started making jewelry from my recovery bed. I sold them for little money. But it was enough to help pay for a few household items.

Later, I was advised to take Sterling to Miami where doctors knew about our disease. So I packed up the jeep and headed south. When we got there Sterling immediately had heart issues and went into C-ICU at the Children's Hospital.

I was still in Miami when one day I got a call from the police in Georgia saying my house had been broken into. Robbers had backed up a truck and took everything we owned right down to my son's toys.

I couldn't leave, my son was too sick. Bank of America then claimed I abandoned the house. They quadrupled my insurance which more than doubled the house payment! Despite efforts to work something out, the bank foreclosed on it. So, my child and I ended up homeless in Miami living in a Jeep with nothing.

RESETTING THE COMPASS

I started to sell jewelry again at the local art festivals and then at a resort. That got us into a motel room and then into a house. That was a major turning point to finally getting long term stability in our lives.

The disease tries to wreak havoc on my body, and I still suffer constant pain. I have trouble standing more than five or ten minutes because the pain is so excruciating.

But I fight through the pain to inspire my son. I can't give up. I have to show Sterling that no matter how disabled you are, you can pick something within your limitations and be a success; even if that means making jewelry from your sick bed.

That day in the hospital when he asked me if he was going to die it broke my heart. He said me, "How will I ever be a cop?" His chronic illness won't let him live that dream. But I want him to know there are many options in life for him. I push myself to be an example for him. So he is the real reason for my personal, spiritual and physical success.

My jewelry business has exploded. My collection has been featured in *People En Espanol,* on *Good Morning America En Espanol,* in *Maxim, GQ magazine*, on the Fox Network, on many local TV shows and abroad in Britain and Africa. Pieces are collected around the world from different art galleries and my online store. You can see my jewelry on the necks of stars like Gloria Gaynor, Lynda Carter, Sandra Bernhard and on the cast of *New Moon*.

In the first half of my life destructive relationships almost ruined me. Now I have a healthy self-image because I took responsibility for my son. It was my fight to protect and care for him since the day he was born that truly changed me. The work to build my business was inspired by him. I cherish our loving relationship and I am on a rewarding journey despite my illness. I had to become strong for my son so that I could raise my miracle child to be a strong, positive man who will hope-fully go on to teach others to be as strong and positive as he is.

JOSETTE REDEFINES WEALTH, HEALTH AND HAPPINESS

I have lived through so many incredible obstacles and have come out successful, positive and happy. I am ready and willing to help everyone else get to their happy place.

I know my purpose is to help others who are stuck in abusive and horrible circumstances. Life has also equipped me to help people who are disabled and have chronic debilitating illnesses and disease. They need to learn how to find their strength and happiness, get on the road to having a fulfilling life, and not be miserable and a victim any longer.

I have a strong and powerful story that I know will motivate others to find their own LeadHERship power. I am here to be of service to God and to thank the universe. I don't look to the past as being bad. It made me who I am. I am a good, strong woman who now loves herself. And I deserve to be happy. So now I build my life on my future, not my past.

POURING LIFE INTO OTHERS

Oh my gosh, it's so much more fun to give than receive. Because of my time on the streets begging for food, I have great compassion for the homeless. I feed the local homeless mostly nice, hot meals. I fill up the back of my truck and go through bushes and try to find the hard to find homeless, just to let them know someone cares.

I have also developed a non-profit called "Dare to Dream a New Reality." We help disabled artists start their own craft business to generate extra money to supplement their disability check and give them a feeling of purpose.

When I first met one of the artists she was in a wheelchair and talked about how she was ready to die. Now she walks with a walker and her jewelry is in stores here in the Florida Keys area, and now she has a smile on her face.

JOSETTE'S TEN RELATIONSHIP TIPS
Loving Yourself First

- Don't allow others to use and abuse you.
- Do not abuse, badger or condemn yourself for your past.
- Know that healing always starts with you, not someone else.
- Learn from past relationships to make future ones better.
- Teach others by sharing your story. It's healing. And it could possibly change someone else's life in the process.
- Don't expect your love to magically heal someone and vice versa; you have to love yourself.
- If you are stuck in an abusive relationship, look at what it's costing you. It's not worth it.
- Harmful relationships suck your life source. Healthy relationships help you live life full of joy and purpose. Know the difference.
- Love the child within. Nurture that child. He or she can do amazing things—just wait and see.
- You are never too old to reinvent yourself and create new, worthy relationships to bless others and broaden you.

Josette Redwolf is wardrobe, jewelry designer and fashion stylist to celebrities and fashion photographers. Learn more about her work and passion at www.josetteredwolf.com.

MY REDEFINING MOMENT
Setting a Better Sail

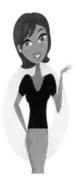

The relationship course Josette Redwolf traveled almost left her shipwrecked at sea. She eventually chose to course-correct. What specific steps can you take to re-define and readjust your relationship with "self" to ensure relationships with others are rich, healthy and produce mutual happiness?

_____

_____

_____

_____

_____

_____

_____

_____

Scholarship

"In learning you will teach, and in teaching you will learn."
~ *Phil Collins*

STAY OUT OF the shallow end of the pool if you want to learn how to dive. High diving, especially, is for serious swimmers; much like focused learning is for serious scholars.

Scholarship is learning at a higher level. Getting there was a grueling climb for Bible scholar Dr. Shirley Cheng. Life itself has been her harshest teacher. Yet she refuses to quit and settle for shallow-water living. Because of that resolve life has been her most rewarding teacher as well.

Dr. Cheng has been wheelchair-bound since she was an infant. The last time she saw a sunset was thirteen years ago. But neither blindness nor disability dims her love of life. Nor have they dulled her desire to "see" the brighter side of her debilitating illness and use it as "teachable moments."

Some see blindness as a curse. Dr. Cheng says she "views" it as a blessing in disguise. She believes it has offered her a unique gift: to truly get to know herself, and forge a stronger relationship with God. She now lives life redefining what wealth, health and happiness look like.

It would be quite easy for Dr. Cheng to "see" her glass half empty. Few people would blame her. But this student of life chooses to "see" her cup full and running over.

For Dr. Cheng, lesson number one on scholarship is quite simple: If you stop learning today you'll start dying tomorrow.

Have you been to the beach lately? Notice how the restless waves anxiously push further inland before the current yanks them back. The human mind also longs to push out further. It desires to explore new territories, uncover hidden truths on earth and beyond.

It's that longing to know which led Christopher Columbus to toss caution to the wind and sail "the ocean blue" in search of the unknown beyond his familiar shores. We humans yearn to learn what's out there, what's inside; what make us tick. And no matter our age or limited ability this natural curiosity is never quite quenched.

Our quest for knowledge makes us rocket into space to explore every dark corner of the universe. And we won't be happy until we touch the face of God. This pursuit feeds our souls. It satisfies our thirst and makes our journey joyful. Why? It gives us meaning.

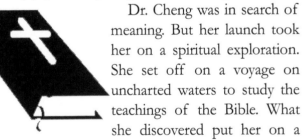

Dr. Cheng was in search of meaning. But her launch took her on a spiritual exploration. She set off on a voyage on uncharted waters to study the teachings of the Bible. What she discovered put her on a lifelong path to follow a plain, but profound fisherman. His words spoken more than two thousand years ago dared her to step out of her boat of limitations. It challenged this blind woman to "see" the world through the eyes of love, gratitude and appreciation… then to go and make disciples.

Dr. Cheng thinks she's found what many curious scholars truly seek: a personal connection to the divine power behind the wonders of life itself, God Almighty.

And that relationship, she says, has brought her peace, purpose and happiness even from her wheelchair; even while being blind.

FLOWING WITH CLEAR VISION
DR. SHIRLEY CHENG

"Although the world is full of suffering, it is full also of the overcoming of it."

~ Helen Keller

I'VE BEEN WHEELCHAIR-BOUND since infancy and blind since age seventeen, yet I'm passionately in love with life!

It might not look that way from the surface, especially during my childhood years.

I was born in 1983. Eleven months later I contracted severe juvenile rheumatoid arthritis after receiving a tuberculin (TB) skin test. I spent my early years in constant pain; some days I was like a statue, unable to move or sit. My mother Juliet Cheng took me to China six times to seek treatment within my first eleven years of life, thus saving my life many times as a result.

Mom lost custody of me twice in the United States only after refusing unwanted and harmful treatments for me; once when I was twenty-two months old and the other time when I was seven.

In 1990 my medical case in Connecticut made international headlines. The doctor wanted to operate on six of my joints in a single operation when he didn't even have any medicine to control my inflammation. Mother wisely said no to the surgery and lost her right to be my parent.

The battle went on for five months. And by the time my mother won, I had become all skin and bones and was vomiting a large amount of blood under his "care," which consisted of administering Naprosyn to me on an empty stomach and frequent x-rays and blood tests.

FACING THE RISING TIDE OF CHALLENGES

Because of years of hospitalization between America and China, I received no education until age eleven. Back then, I only knew my ABCs and very little English; other than that, my book knowledge was non-existent. So I started elementary school in a special education class. After only 180 days I had mastered the grade levels so well I was immediately moved to regular 6th grade in middle school. I had a passion for learning and received numerous academic awards. I was Student of the Year in 6th grade, Student of the Month in 7th grade, and got an excellence award for achieving the highest grade for Earth science in the entire 8th grade class.

I was a top honor student, being on the Principal's List several times in high school. I also contributed to my high school newspaper as an artist. I ran for student body vice president as a freshman, and received a standing ovation for my platform speech as a candidate.

NO SIGHT, BUT CLEAR VISION

I lost my eyesight at age seventeen, but that did not stop me from loving the life I live. It did stop me from attending school though, so I received home-tutoring instead. I completed my schoolwork using only cassette tapes and recorded my assignments, like essays, for teachers to grade at school.

Even with a three-point nine GPA I couldn't accumulate enough credits to graduate. So I earned my GED instead. I took the entire GED test, including mathematical calculations and problem solving, graphs, and an essay, in my head without Braille; (I can't use Braille because of my severe juvenile rheumatoid arthritis)

Because of my arthritis, I can type with only my two index fingers, but I can produce about sixty-five words per minute. And by age twenty, I became an author, completing three books within one year. Now at age thirty, I'm an award-winning author with twenty-seven book awards. I've written nine books and contributed to twenty-five, as well as being an editor of one.

Did I mention that I love learning? In 2010, I earned my doctorate in Divinity as a summa cum laude graduate.

DIVINE ENLIGHTENMENT

I am constantly expanding my knowledge in the Word of God by studying the Bible and teaching what I've learned to those who are eager to take in God's Word as refreshing water.

I had always been more than curious about the Bible, but never had a chance to read it. After I lost my sight I gained all the time in the world. Thus, my journey in deepening my relationship with God began. I was nineteen when I read the Bible for the first time. Since then,

I've read it fourteen more times, using twelve different versions.

Knowing God fulfills my curiosity about life. It answers the most pivotal questions: Where have I come from? Why am I here? Where will I go? How can I live the best life possible? The Bible is the ultimate life's manual. It is the map and compass I use to guide me on the right path to living a positive life that harmonizes with God's will.

WADING THROUGH THE WHYS

Why I contracted juvenile rheumatoid arthritis at eleven months old or why I lost my eyesight at age seventeen, or why I experienced all other challenges in between: these are questions I have no answers to. But I do know that challenges are life's vaccines: they equip your soul with the necessary tools to battle future storms. They strengthen my faith in God and develop in me enduring qualities, just as the Bible says: "*We rejoice in hope of the glory of God. Not only this, but we also rejoice in our sufferings, knowing that suffering works perseverance; and perseverance, proven character; and proven character, hope; and hope doesn't disappoint us, because God's love has been poured out into our hearts through the Holy Spirit who was given to us.*" (Romans 5:2-5, WEB)

If there were no darkness, how could the stars appear so bright? If there were no challenges, how could I name myself a victor?

Moreover, I see the loss of my eyesight as a divine turn of events. While God didn't actually cause my blindness, He did bless me with a new spiritual vision in place of my physical sight. I now am better able to steer my life in the right or better direction, as I have Yahweh's everlasting principles to guide and lead me.

A WAVE OF PASSION

If I hadn't lost my eyesight, I would have become a scientist as I had hoped. I wanted to be a scientist to find the cures to some of the deadliest diseases. But the thing is: even if we can discover cures to all known diseases, we cannot offer people eternal life--only God can, through obedience to His will and faith in Jesus Christ.

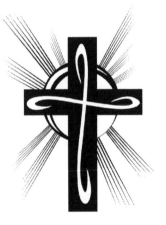

Now as a Bible teacher I can introduce people to the ultimate healer. I get to teach the entire Bible in depth, from Genesis to Revelation, one-on-one via e-mail. I have students from around the world who work on my Bible lessons, complete assignments and take tests. Yes, I write all my lessons and tests from scratch.

Leave it to God to squeeze my lemons into refreshing lemonade for His glory! For the first time in my life, I feel I've found my purpose of existence. For the first time, I have sight of where I'm headed, and most importantly, that I'm heading in the right direction, for there's no better guidance than that from my very Life-Giver.

I'm living the life of my wildest dream, a life I never imagined I would be privileged enough to live, a life that I hope will transcend duty, beyond mere humanly accomplishments, to a life of service for the betterment of humanity.

DR. CHENG REDEFINES WEALTH, HEALTH AND HAPPINESS

The greatest wealth anyone can attain in life is a sacred relationship with our Creator, God Almighty.

Let's consider material wealth for a moment. We can have absolutely everything we want in life: huge mansions, fancy cars, ever-expanding wardrobes, and a sailboat or two to boot. But should our lives be measured by monetary values? Is the worth of our lives so calculable that we can consider ourselves wealthy simply by adding up our material possessions?

Even if we feel wealthy by owning great possessions, what good would such wealth do us when natural calamities take them away from us? And when we die, could we take our wealth to our graves? Thus, *our lives shouldn't "consist of the abundance of the things* [we possess]." (Luke 12:15, WEB)

So, true wealth is being rich toward God Almighty, the very Creator who has given us the precious gift of life. Being rich toward God is establishing and maintaining a sacred and intimate relationship with Him and His Son by walking according to God's will and laws. Such a relationship will never grow old; it'll be *"a treasure in the heavens that doesn't fail, where no thief approaches, neither moth destroys."* (Luke 12:33) Such a treasure is immeasurable.

COUNTING THE BLESSINGS

Life has taught me to be happy and appreciate the journey. I have learned to be content in whatever situation I'm in. I have lost my eyesight and the ability to walk; yet, I'm never scornful. Instead, I'm simply grateful for having owned these powers before. Plus, I am still the owner of so many other wonderful gifts; I can still talk, I can still hear, and I am still alive, so I utilize all these great factors to become an award-winning author and a motivational speaker to touch as many people as I possibly can to bring humor, hope, and healing.

I am so privileged to know, discover, and experience all the wonderful things life has to offer. I am able to laugh; I am able to weep. Without my existence, I would be able to do none of these. Why should I resist all the wonders of life just because negativity decides to bump into me? Compared to the entire universe and all the beauties it contains, my problems are tiny! God gave me my life so I can enjoy it to its fullest, and this is exactly what I will always do.

Although I'm blind, I can see far and wide; even though I'm disabled, I can climb high mountains. I let the ropes of hope in God haul me high!

DR. CHENG'S TEN SCHOLARSHIP TIPS

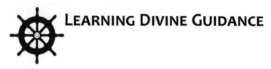 **LEARNING DIVINE GUIDANCE**

- Revere and love your Creator. It opens your heart to learn valuable lessons of life

- Seize every opportunity to learn. Grab every chance you have to learn a new subject or take up a new hobby, for if you wait for the "perfect moment" or the "right opportunity," it may never come.

- Be receptive to constructive criticism. If you love correction, you love knowledge (Proverbs 12:1). To receive and learn from constructive criticism is wisdom, for you'll gain better understanding: *"The ear that listens to reproof lives, and will be at home among the wise…"*

- Take lessons from nature. From God's beautiful creations, learn to be: diligent in storing up for the future as the ants, driven and hardworking as the bees, and devoted as a pair of loons. Diligence, a driven will, and devotion are the keys to a good learner, as *"in all hard work there is profit."* (Proverbs 14:23, WEB)

- Be swift to hear, slow to speak. Among the first steps in attaining wisdom is to listen. To soak up knowledge, carefully listen to instruction with attentive ears without interrupting, for *"whoever despises instruction will pay for it, but he who respects a command will be rewarded."* (Proverbs 13:13, WEB)

- Embrace humility to absorb knowledge. Pride holds us back from listening to the instruction, advice, and suggestions of others. Only humility will allow you to receive instruction and consider suggestions with an open heart, and that will lead you to wisdom, for the *"way of a fool is right in his own eyes, but he who is wise listens to counsel."* (Proverbs 12:15, WEB)

- Realize the value of knowledge. If you understand and acknowledge that "wisdom is better than rubies" and "all the things that may be desired can't be compared to it," then you will be motivated and empowered to seek after *"instruction rather than silver; knowledge rather than choice gold."* (Proverbs 8:10-11, WEB)

- Learn from your mistakes. Failure is not the result of our mistakes; failure is the outcome when we have failed to learn from our mistakes. To improve your walk in life, learn from your past to see how you can do things differently to attain better results.

- Learn from the aged. There is wisdom and insight in age and experience. As the Chinese proverb says, "The older the ginger, the hotter the spice." Do not hesitate to seek the counsel of your parents, grandparents, or trusted older friends. Their experience in life may provide you with the insights you need. Remember, *"Where there is no counsel, plans fail; but in a multitude of counselors they are established.*" (Proverbs 15:22, WEB)

- Apply your knowledge to your life. Obtaining knowledge is merely the beginning of learning, not something at which you should stop. What good is your knowledge if you do not apply it to your life? Application of your knowledge is "learning through experience."

Dr. Shirley Cheng is Bible Teacher, Gospel Proclaimer, Award-winning Author, Motivational Speaker, Poet and Founder of www.Ultra-Ability.com Ministry

My Redefining Moment

Setting a Better Sail

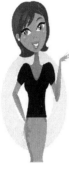

Scholarship demands higher-level learning. Self-improvement starts with spiritual improvement. How much time do you set aside to read, reflect and connect with God? What steps can you take to develop a habit of feeding your faith?

_____

_____

_____

_____

_____

_____

_____

Stewardship

Life is a gift, and it offers us the privilege, opportunity, and responsibility to give something back by becoming more."
~ *Anthony Robbins*

So, JUST HOW does a homeless teenager in a foreign country become a celebrated self-made millionaire?

Ask Shanna McFarlane. She is founder and CEO of a multi-million dollar Global Real Estate Investment company headquartered in Toronto, Canada. Last year, she was nominated for the Woman Entrepreneur of the Year award. She was cited as one of the most powerful women in real estate investing.

Shanna knows what it's like to hob-knob with the wise and wealthy. She also knows how it feels to be homeless, hungry and desperate enough to beg for food. Her gritty story of rejection, struggle and rapid climb to wealth reads like a Cinderella tale, but without Prince Charming.

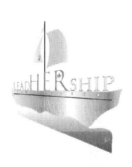

In 1994, Shanna immigrated to Canada from the West Indies in search of a better life. Instead, her world turned upside down. She ended up on the streets, sleeping in airport terminals and pan-handling outside a supermarket.

Shanna's father and stepmom in Canada had sponsored her move there. She said they mistreated her when she arrived, later withdrew their support and left her to fend for herself.

But Shanna had fire in her belly, and trouble only stoked the embers. She was determined to survive. She was also destined to succeed no matter how much failure flaunted itself in her face. It was just a matter of time before she found her footing.

Like so many people who bear the mark of greatness Shanna had a gift that the world had to make room for. First she had to discover this natural ability and then steward it well.

Stewardship is the care and protection of one's skills and talents to use in the service of others. It also means to manage another person's property.

Each of us is born with a unique gift. Some people say our gifts are talents on loan from God. And we steward or manage His "property" well when we nurture them, master them and use them to uplift and empower others.

A person who excels in a particular field is called gifted. History considers pianist Ludwig Van Beethoven a gifted composer. But such a gift seldom comes wrapped in pretty packaging. Beethoven's most famous works were composed when he was almost totally deaf. Often it's tragedy, struggle or distress that stirs up a person's gift or pushes it into the realm of greatness.

Such was the case with Shanna. She is naturally gifted or skilled in business, particularly real estate acquisitions.

It was her own struggle with poverty that put her on the road to wealth. Difficulties made her develop the drive that helped reveal and refine her gift.

It's a gift that keeps on giving as an example of perseverance, purpose and self- determination.

Cast Your Bread upon the Water

By Shanna McFarlane

> *"God prospers me not to raise my standard of living, but to raise my standard of giving."*
>
> ~ *Randy Alcorn*

HERE I WAS, alone aboard a plane headed back to Canada on a one-way ticket. That's when it hit me like a punch to the stomach: where would I go once the plane lands? I had no idea. I was so busy trying to get back in the country I hadn't thought that far ahead.

When reality kicked in I started to panic. I was nervous, scared but oddly enough, still a bit excited about having the opportunity to return to Canada.

My mind started racing. The thought of how my father just left me in another country made me furious all over again. I felt abandoned. I watched as everyone who got off my flight had someone waiting at the arrival gate for them, except me!

For hours I sat in the airport lobby in a bewildered daze. By midnight the airport security guards had asked me more than ten times, "Mam, are you ok?" "I'm fine," I said, "Just waiting for a postponed flight." Thank God my height made me look much older than my age of sixteen.

I had less than sixty dollars in my purse and I knew that wasn't enough for a hotel. Even if it was, what would I do after that? I felt as if my world just kept crumbling around me and I could do no right.

And for the first time I actually started to feel that my dad was right about me; maybe I was "useless" after all. Soon my brain hit the replay button, and the memories flooded my mind.

FIGHTING EARLY HEADWINDS

I was born and grew up in the beautiful Island of Jamaica. My parents split when I was quite young, so my mom raised me. My dad migrated to Canada, remarried and started a family there. When I was fifteen, he sponsored me to come to Canada to live with him and his new family. I was excited for the opportunity, but still nervous. I had never lived with my dad, plus now we had a new family in the mix. Nonetheless, I said my goodbyes and I was off to Canada.

When I got to Canada I knew this wasn't going to be easy. I felt I could do nothing right. It seems I was always in trouble for something and the entire family made it clear I was not a welcome guest!

To me it appeared obvious my dad took me out of obligation and didn't really want me. And my stepmom made it painfully clear she did not want a stepchild.

After four months there I was dreadfully home sick and constantly punished for one thing or the other. My dad and stepmom would complain about how much food I ate. They always seemed to insinuate that I was dumb and gave me the impression that my mom in Jamaica did a poor job raising me. When they went out as a family I was often left home. There was no doubt in my mind I was the unloved and unwanted black sheep.

RIPPLES OF DECEPTION

One day my dad told me we were going on vacation for a week in Jamaica to visit my grandmother who was ill. I was excited to go because I had a lot on my plate and it would be good to see my mom and grandmother.

When we got to Jamaica however, my dad called a family meeting and told me he was not taking me back with him. This was his plot all along. My grandmother was not ill and this was not a vacation. I felt he had tricked me in order to take me back. My dad not only left me behind in Jamaica he also took my passport with my visa back to Canada. That was his way of ensuring I would not return.

I was humiliated, angry, hurt and devastated to say the least. My entire family was in an uproar. No one except a few asked me what happened. Instead they blamed me and demanded, "How could you have screwed up such an opportunity?"

For months I called dad and stepmom every day, begging them to return my passport. Many times they answered the phone and told me not to call back, then hung up. I was stuck. Here I was, a fifteen year-old living with friends; out of school, no job, no money, no direction, no hope and no future by the looks of it!

A DIVE OF DESPERATION

About six months later, I muscled up my last ounce of courage and decided to go to the Canadian Visa office in Jamaica. I had planned on telling the immigration officer a lie; that I had lost my passport and my visa. At the time lying made sense. I was too ashamed to say my dad had abandoned me. The truth, I thought, would certainly have people thinking I must be a bad person, and no one would want to help.

As I sat down and the officer asked me why I was there, my mind went completely blank. I just stared into space. For the life of me, I couldn't remember the story I had planned to tell.

That's when the tears came like a flood. I remember crying as if my mother had just died, I let everything out. All the emotions I had kept inside for so long came surging out. The officer let me cry without interruption. Once I was able to compose myself, I told her the whole story, the ugly truth about the last six months.

That day that immigration officer not only gave me a one-way visa back to Canada but she gave me inspiration that reset the course of my life. She said, "Don't ever let someone else's opinion of you determine who you are and how far you can go!" On that note I was on my way back to Toronto.

SENDING OUT AN SOS

So, there I was spending the night in the airport lobby in a corner, quietly crying and silently praying. I would spend two nights there moving from one terminal to another so the airport security guards wouldn't get suspicious.

In the middle of my pity party and feeling sick to my stomach, I remembered I had met one girl in school who had befriended me. But she hadn't heard from me in almost six months and I was too embarrassed to have to explain my situation. How I even remembered her phone number is a miracle. But I finally mustered the courage and made the call. She was so excited to hear my voice and when I told her what had happened to me, she did not hesitate to help. The next day she sent me a one-way Greyhound bus ticket to her home in Ottawa. Just like that I was on my way... on my way to start a new chapter.

TROUBLING STORMS

A few years went by and I was on my own and doing ok. At least my life was on track. I was going to school and working when the city transit went on strike. Ordinarily this wouldn't be a big deal. But when you are working minimum wage and you don't have a car, your savings dry up pretty quickly. Within a few months I was behind on my rent and soon evicted from my home. I sought refuge at a shelter. To stay there and get help I was told, by law, I had to accept welfare. But that posed a big moral dilemma.

Here was an opportunity to get back at my dad and stepmom for abandoning me. Under immigration laws I could accept social assistance. But my sponsors would have to repay the government all the money I got if they ever wanted to sponsor another family member.

Now I hadn't talked with my family since returning to Canada. I was still bitterly angry at them for treating me so viciously. But I knew I had a stepbrother in Jamaica whom my dad and stepmom planned to sponsor. I also knew they could never afford to repay any money I took from the government. Even though I was still furious, I turned down the social assistance for their sake. Needless to say I was evicted from the shelter. And just like that I was homeless.

The months that followed were very difficult. Some of my lowest points came when I had to stand outside a grocery store and beg shoppers for a dollar just so I could eat.

FINDING FORGIVENESS

It took me awhile to get my life together, because for years I refused to "own" or take full responsibility for my life. I felt I was wronged by the people who were supposed to be there for me. And forgiving them was hard. For several years I continued to struggle financially and emotionally. Then I realized I not only had to forgive my past, but embrace my story; for it was a gift. And that mind shift eventually helped push me into purpose and destiny.

Somehow I knew I was born to do something great and make a big difference in the world. I was never satisfied with just working for someone else. I wanted to own something. I always had an entrepreneurial streak. Even on my lowest days I was giving business advice to someone.

A GIVING SPIRIT

I remember on one job, if you sat at my table during the lunch break the conversation always steered toward business and entrepreneurship. My colleagues always came to me for financial and business advice even when I didn't have money. They always said I was a natural entrepreneur and would ask, "Why are you wasting time here?"

When I brought up the topic of launching or growing a business, most would say "I don't know what kind of business to start," or "I don't know anything about business." I often simplified it and showed them how to monetize their hobbies and turn them into profitable businesses.

I remember a colleague who was very passionate about baking. She would always bring us treats. One day I sat down with her and showed her how to differentiate herself in the marketplace by making and marketing treats for diabetics. She has since launched a full business making diabetic treats.

Another colleague was studying esthetics part-time. I advised her not to look for a job in the field but to start her own business. I made a business and marketing plan for her. I lso showed her how to specialize in her industry and do what other spas weren't doing. She used the business plan I created and got funding for her first day spa. Last I heard she now owns three spas in the USA and Columbia.

All this before I even started a business consulting company! It wasn't long after that I started to take my own advice.

LEAPING INTO SUCCESS

I started to read and research anything I could on people who were successful: those who had achieved financial greatness. What I discovered was they all had real estate and business in common. So, I decided to simply follow their lead to success. I wasted no time and jumped head-long into real estate. I never looked back.

At age twenty-nine I started my real estate investing company, and in just eighteen months I had a multi-million dollar empire. Since then several other companies have sprung up. I started a beauty supply chain from the trunk of my car with only two hundred dollars. Then I opened a business consulting firm for entrepreneurs looking to grow.

At sixteen I was homeless, by thirty-one I was a millionaire. I have been a good steward over the business gift God had given me.

In 2012, I was nominated for the Woman Entrepreneur of the Year. Several years ago, an international magazine chose me as one of the most influential female real estate investors and entrepreneurs in North America. When I got the call with the news I panicked. I was always afraid of being seen as a victim, even though I had come so far and done so much.

But I again realized my "rags to riches" story was my gift to the world. And sharing it was my responsibility as a good steward. After that magazine hit the newsstands I was inundated with e-mails from people who said they were inspired and empowered by my journey "From Homeless to Millionaire."

SHANNA REDEFINES WEALTH, HEALTH AND HAPPINESS

For me, wealth is the ability to use your story, experience, knowledge and purpose to inspire and influence others. More importantly, it's the ability to empower people to plug into their higher calling on their personal and professional life journey.

One of the things I've learned on my journey is that no one but you can take ownership for your life and business. I am at the helm. And I "lead my ship" by taking full responsibility and being accountable for the outcome and results in my life. While doing this I've been able to inspire, empower and lead others who aspire to achieve success. And that has brought me much joy.

My happiness comes from the satisfaction of using and improving my gift, and in giving back. I mentor women and young entrepreneurs through workshops, speaking at organizations and hosting my own seminars and providing scholarships to certain events.

Without my early struggles I would have missed out on the opportunity to help change and improve lives. I would have missed out on inspiring hope!

Just about every day I receive emails from people describing how I've impacted the way they now think about business and about life. I have had the great pleasure of lifting so many others as I climb.

BE THE GIFT

Now I know everything in life happens for a purpose and no experience goes wasted, even the heart-wrenching ones.

Yes, my story is my gift to the world! I have realized that God chose me because He knew I was strong enough to endure, to fight through with tenacity, to persevere with grace and share my life with humility!

I believe most of us have a seed in our hearts to soar. But for various reasons we choose to crawl. The truth is when a vision is rooted in you for something great you must never consent to anything less.

That's even more sobering when you realize that many lives hinge on you caring for your great gift.

Your good stewardship will inspire them to create their own greatness.

SHANNA'S TEN STEWARDSHIP TIPS
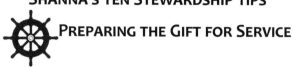
PREPARING THE GIFT FOR SERVICE

- Know that life is God's gift to you. Live it as a gift to others.
- Take ownership for your life and business. You are your best steward.
- Nurture yourself in order to nurture others. The giver must replenish.
- Always make time to inspire and empower. The more you teach the more you learn.
- Don't be afraid to tell your story of struggle to triumph. Lives will be changed.
- Manage the little things well. This leads to greatness.
- Serve from a place of love, service and humility. People can spot a fake.
- Tithe your talent into your community. Help build the world you desire.
- Expect to face obstacles. They can become your strengthening tool.
- Discover ways to add value. Do more than people expect.

Shanna McFarlane is known as the Power-house Entrepreneur who went from "Homeless on the Streets to Owning the Street!" She owns and operates a multi-million dollar real estate empire in Toronto, Canada. www.shannamcfarlane.com

MY REDEFINING MOMENT

SETTING A BETTER SAIL

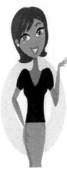

We all came to the planet equipped with gifts or special skills. They are seeds we plant in the garden of life. It's our responsibility to nurture them, to use them well to serve ourselves and serve humanity. That is good stewardship. What is your gift and how do you work to perfect it? How is it making a difference in people's lives?

_____

_____

_____

_____

_____

_____

_____

_____

PART II
SET YOURSELF UP
FOR SUCCESS

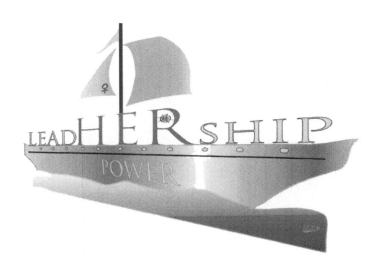

When Women Rock the Boat

"I didn't get there by wishing for it or hoping for it, but by working for it."

~ Estee Lauder

MORE WOMEN ARE bolting for the exit doors of corporate America. They are choosing to chart their own course as entrepreneurs. According to Forbes magazine, "In the past decade the number of privately owned businesses started by women in the U.S. has increased twice as fast as the number owned by men."

Working nine-to-five to build someone's dreams is taking a back seat to sailing solo and being the captain of your own ship. And with the surge of business start-ups by women comes a redefining of what business looks like.

Profit margins are not just gauged in dollars and cents. The definition of wealth now extends to the ability to make a valuable difference. Much stock is put in currencies that might weigh less on Wall Street; currencies like compassion, faith, community service driven by a sense of purpose.

This LeadHERship Power is anchored on exceptional business talent, skill, dedication and experience. It's also rooted in intuition, emotion and heart-driven feminine sensibility. It's something former top business executive Lucy Hoger relied on to successfully navigate her male-dominated business environment before launching her own ship.

Saving a Sinking Ship

"If you want something said, ask a man. If you want something done, ask a woman."- Margaret Thatcher,

~ Former British Prime Minister

THE INTRACTABLE FORMER British Prime Minister, Margaret Thatcher, made that blunt statement above. It no doubt troubled the waters among her staunch male critics in Parliament. Women around the world likely took it as a delightful confirmation of the obvious.

It describes business strategist Lucy Hoger quite well. She was once a Price Waterhouse consultant handling high-end projects for big oil companies like Exxon, Shell, Arco and Amoco. During the early stages of the dot-com boom in the late 1990's, Hoger gave herself a demotion and moved to Silicon Valley as a project manager for a start-up internet company.

The company was an early version of eBay. And Hoger was the executive in charge of the services organization that implemented the software.

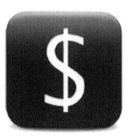

In three years the company went public and raised about $150 million. Hoger said, "Over the course of those three years, three different CEOs went through all of the money and departed. We were left as a company with only $5 million."

Worried investors were ready to jump ship and call it quits as the company faced bankruptcy. But as it began to collapse, Hoger took charge. She convinced the Board of Directors to give her and the remaining engineering team a chance to save the failing business.

"I said, I am now declaring myself the new Chief Operating Officer of this company and here's the deal: There are only 30 of us left. Allow us to stay open. Allow us to use the $5 million. And in twenty-four to forty-eight months, we will either declare bankruptcy or we will sell the company [at a profit]. I was that confident. I knew we could go up against the odds and actually create a new product, get new customers and create such a buzz in the market-place that we could do this."

"And we did it! We literally said we're going to own it.

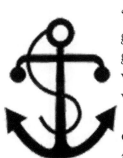

We're going to have an attitude of 'failure is not an option' and we're going to get creative about it. We're going to have fun. And just because we're the underdogs doesn't mean we're supposed to lose."

"As employees, we're leading our company. The competition was liter-ally calling us losers because they were going on to more fun and exciting technologies. That was when Silicon Valley was really, really buzzing. And we just said, you know what, one of these days, we're going to be the ones on top. We're going to be making that phone call and say, 'Well, while you were gone, this is what we accomplished.'

"As I predicted, because I knew what the customers needed, we actually were able to turn the company around. We created a competitive war between two companies, one of them being IBM, to the tune where we sold the business for $90 million."

Hoger showed her LeadHERship chops when she led the charge and pulled the company back from the brink of bankruptcy. And she did it in a high-stakes, male-dominated marketplace. She pulled it off, thanks to years of experience and stellar work as an innovative strategist. But she also pulled on her feminine sensibility and intuition.

BE A CRUSADER

Few people will disagree with the notion that women are more intuitive than men. Women tend to lead from the heart as well as the head. So, apparently, it was not enough for Hoger to acknowledge that what the former CEOs did to suck the company dry was wrong. Somehow she felt obligated to right that wrong.

"The thing you always have to remember is that to men business is a chess game. It's not about emotion. It's simply about winning the game.

Typically to women, it's about saving face, self and core. So as long as I understand that, the question becomes how can I save face? We've gotten ourselves into a really tough situation. There's an integrity part of this, and integrity becomes very important for businesswomen who are high-end executives. To them if the core is cracked it doesn't matter what's on the business agenda. If that integrity is broken, you've got to repair integrity first, business second."

"So, let's go back to the $5 million I turned into $90 million. How did I do that? Well, because I knew there was a better way and that better way turned into a crusade. It tuned into a crusade because we just said, 'this is wrong,' and nobody would listen to us. So we just went in and decided to be mavericks."

"I think it's important that you have a crusade. People call it different things; a cause, a purpose."

Whatever you call it, Hoger says women who desire to lead their business or personal lives with conviction and purpose must be clear about it. And they must have a boat-load of confidence.

Clarity comes from knowing your "why." So why are you getting in there and fighting for (your cause) so much?

Confidence is what you need in the face of adversity. You'll face adversity when you really want to play at a much higher level.

Hoger was bold enough to take the helm of her sinking dot-com ship because of her conviction. She knew the right thing to do was to correct a wrong. She provided strategic LeadHERship to course-correct. That move generated a surge of cash flow that rescued her company.

Launch Out into Deep Waters

Lucy Hoger's 13 Business Success Strategies

If you are ready to take the plunge as a new business owner or want to sure up your entrepreneurial skills, here are thirteen business strategies Lucy Hoger offers to help you set yourself up for success:

⚓ *Prepare your Mindset*

Mindset is about your BIG WHY. Being an entrepreneur requires a personal dedication that you can, and will, make a difference with the gifts you have to share with the world. That conviction comes from seeing things in unique ways that others overlook. If I can help just one person or one business, that's just as satisfying to me as helping many. Helping that one person or business creates a ripple effect for so many others who may remain unknown to me. And if their lives are truly improved, they will find me through referrals. What a great opportunity to create countless ripples in the world!

⚓ Position Yourself as an Expert

An expert is a person who has a comprehensive and authoritative knowledge of a skill or strategy in a particular area. My unique experience and perspective doing corporate turn-arounds in

Silicon Valley allows me to be an expert in business strategy. Defining my experience in a quantitative manner quickly establishes credibility with business people. They respond to numbers which paint a picture of success in their mind. Coupling these numbers with my experience in helping businesses quickly overcome their customer and internal challenges, this completes the picture of expertise accompanied with demonstrated results.

⚙ Shift from Worker to Business Owner

First build confidence in your own ability. It's impossible to become a successful business owner without it. In Maslow's hierarchy of needs theory, the pinnacle of the pyramid is self-actualization for creativity, spontaneity and problem solving. This pinnacle is reached when one's self-esteem, confidence, achievement, respect of others and by others have been realized. Study Maslow's hierarchy. This is the best framework available that shows the mind shift from worker to business owner.

⚙ Create a New Career from Past Experience

Creating a new career around your years of experience can be both exciting and frightening all at the same time. It's exciting because you are the expert and have a unique view about solving business problems based on what has worked time and time again for you.

It's frightening when measuring your expertise against the numerous professionals who are also experts. Fighting off that little voice of self-doubt inside you is as great a challenge as any outside threat to the new business. At the end of the day, it's THE most empowering feeling when you finally tell yourself, "I've got this."

Save Before You Walk Away

For the majority of entrepreneurs transitioning from a "regular" job, it's best to start the business while being employed. By starting the venture on a part-time basis you can work out the kinks in your business. Reduce your recurring debt as much as possible as well as your personal living expense while the new business is gaining momentum. This is a critical part of being in business for yourself. Managing expenses is as important as generating revenue (cash). If you have lower expenses, reaching your profitability threshold is reduced.

Now that you are lean and mean you're ready to think about how much to save for the future. The savings must not only cover your living expenses but the on-going development and expansion of your business, plus an unexpected contingency fund.

Take time to create an honest budget for both your living expenses as well as your business for the next year. Whatever number is arrived at during this exercise add 30 percent for the unknown. Most businesses fail within five years of starting due to underfunding. Without the budgeting process, you will be guessing your way to financial difficulty. Poor planning is why so many entrepreneurs take on a part-time job or limp back to the workforce. Don't be that guy.

If you're not good at budgets, recognize that this is part of any successful business. Find an expert (could be a friend who will tell you the truth) who can help you create an effective budget. Being in business for yourself does not mean *by yourself*. Leveraging other people's expertise is needed to be successful.

Maintain and Leverage Old Relationships

People who know and trust you are golden to your business. They wear a number of hats along your path to success: advisors, friendly shoulder to lean on, sounding board that will tell you the truth when you're not going in the right direction. These people know your dreams, aspiration and what's truly in your heart and will help in whatever way they can to see you succeed. Don't forget to reciprocate their generosity.

Invest in Partnership, Synergy, Collaboration

When you're a business owner, you need to have other experts on board that will enhance the experience for your customers. A virtual team is needed to quickly grow your business.

Having experts available in different areas of your business gives you leverage and can transform a sole proprietor into a virtual corporation. Your customers, of course, are looking for your services and products. But they want much more. Once they trust you, they may want recommendations on a range of problems that may require outside help. Your professional network is as important as the expertise you bring to the table. Time is THE most important asset each of us wants more of. If you can offer a quick resolution or answer your customers' needs they will become your raving fans.

Prepare for Rainy Days

Rainy days are part of the journey. Be prepared in four fronts to help quickly shift into a better tomorrow: (1) emotionally, (2) physically, (3) logically and (4) financially. Of the four the most important is to have emotional support from friends and family.

Sometimes we just need to talk about the situation with someone who cares and the solution to the problem mystically presents itself. A family member who knows little about the business can often ask THE most insightful questions that can shift your thinking toward quick resolution to your problem(s). Rainy days can live on in one's mind and magnify in intensity, or can be used to bring about a positive change in the direction of your business. It's your choice.

Physical activity, even if it's going for a long walk, does clear the mind on rainy days. You can release so much of negative energy which will help let you see things more clearly.

Apply logic by writing or journaling your difficulties. Determine the real problem versus the symptom of the problem. Once you know the real problem, create three to five options on how to resolve the situation. The more options the greater the freedom in finding a solution.

Be careful, financial pressures may drive to illogical conclusions. It's key to know your financial limits before acts of desperation take place.

Stay Confident when Business Stalls

Leaders like Gandhi and Martin Luther King continued in the face of adversity because their WHY, their conviction, their purpose transcended the obstacles they faced. It was their inner voice that guided them to greatness. Each of us has that same gift. Your "little voice" will guide you through troubled times when it's not trying to instill doubt. It may tell you to continue on believing that you will succeed. It may tell you to adjust your course in order to succeed. Or it may tell you to take the learning from this business venture to create something new that your customer wants. Staying confident is about knowing in your heart of hearts that you're on the right course: doing what you were meant to do.

Prepare for this day well in advance. When you have success, no matter how small, write yourself a letter of encouragement. You know what you want to hear and what needs to be said in those difficult moments. You'll be amazed at your own wisdom.

Harness the Feeling of Being the Boss

Business owners are an elite group of pioneers who will blaze the trail to prosperity no matter what the economic cycle is doing. We are unique in the world and celebrate the freedoms we have in this country. When we provide jobs for others, placing food on their tables, we take on the needs of our extended "family." For the most part, business owners really care about their customers and employees. We really do want to make the world a better place than we found it. That's what working for yourself really means.

Be Flexible, Adaptable to Change

In the beginning, new ideas keep constantly popping up. Course corrections are part of the discovery process. It's fun, exciting, invigorating and makes you feel alive. At times it can be overwhelming. This is the beginning of The Emotional Cycle of

Change. It's known as Uninformed Optimism.

The next phase of the cycle of change is Informed Pessimism. This phase will determine if you continue or give up. What you're experiencing is completely natural. Every business owner goes through this peak and valley possibly more often than they would like. There's a fine line between giving up and creating a course adjustment. Here's where your self-talk is paramount. Don't listen to the "little voice" that says quit.

That's why it's important to have a business plan with the logical pieces laid out to help balance the emotional reaction to a business adjustment with logical proof. Don't let emotion destroy your dream. Evolve!

Three key factors to keep in mind about being in business are: (1) It's never too late to do the right thing no matter what the circumstances or passage of time. (2) Turn failures into stepping stones by learning what needs to be done better, what needs to be abandoned and what needs to be adopted. (3) Business always undergoes reinvention, and sooner that you think.

Become part of a mastermind group to stay accountable for your actions. More importantly, they can give you encouragement and a fresh perspective when you think the worst is about to happen. Consider joining Sharon Frame's "Focus and Follow Through" mastermind group at www. sharonframespeaks.com.

Don't Be Stressed by Deadlines

A deadline to "making it" assumes failure. Highly successful individuals in history were driven by a sense of purpose. Thomas Edison once stated: "I have not failed. I've just found 10,000 ways that won't work."

It is *purpose* that gives success the legs to get up and run again after a fall. The beauty of a new venture is that you get to redefine how to achieve the outcome. It's the discovery along the way that creates excitement along the journey. "Making it" often does not look like the image that was conceived at the beginning. "Making it" is more about learning along the way about how things work to make things better and to ultimately be of worth to others.

 ## Develop a Daily Success Routine

When starting a new venture, divide the year into quarters with the following objectives:

First Quarter: Learn from experts. Read as much as you can on the topic. Model the habits and behaviors of leaders. Become a student of the subject and have a clear goal of what areas you need to master. Keep a notebook and reference your sources.

Second Quarter: Place into practice what you have learned. Be willing to fail; but fail quickly. This may create an uncomfortable situation of vulnerability and embarrassment at times. Do it anyway. It's through practice and learning from mistakes that will hone your mastery of the subject.

Third Quarter: Study why *success* is being achieved. Understand how people are gaining momentum. Measure quantitatively what has been accomplished.

Fourth Quarter: Celebrate success! Document new concepts and techniques that make you the master in your field. Teach others what you learned and help them master what you know.

Daily routines are aligned to the quarterly objective. Success is messy: some days will be great, some days will be so-so, some days will be a waste. That's OK! Success is achieved through a number of small steps, strung together, along the way to your goal. The key is to keep moving forward no matter what. Small steps consistently made over time create huge results.

LUCY REDEFINES WEALTH, HEALTH AND HAPPINESS

"To *thine* own self be true." "As the man thinketh so is he." William Shakespeare, James Allen and others speak of "being present". Show up every day with your "A GAME," wealth will be a by-product.

Wealth can be defined in so many different ways. Money is only one way of keeping score. Wealth can also be intangible, such as, a great marriage, loving family, caring neighbors, belonging to a spiritually rich church, just to name a few. If you only keep score with money, you may be setting yourself up for disappointment later in life.

Now that I work for myself, happiness, health and wealth take on a different meaning. When I worked for a corporation, I completely focused on the company, employees, customers, and our shareholders. Serving at the pleasure and employment of others becomes a consuming way of life. Now that I'm my own boss, it's about being true to who I am and what I was meant to contribute while on this earth. There is a huge difference in what drives my life. It's who you are, or become on the way to serving others in your life's journey, that creates happiness and health. Reinvent yourself, frequently. It will keep you young!

Health cannot be achieved without happiness. In fact, they're co-dependent. Health starts with who you think you are and what you strive to become. Everyday I'm grateful for what I have and who is in my life. Nutrition and exercise will support the body. But it needs gratitude and happiness to truly excel.

Happiness starts with being comfortable with who you are. Forgiveness is another major piece: seeking forgiveness from others and forgiving yourself. The latter is the hardest to achieve when a terrible event from the past is replayed over and over in your mind, always asking the question: "What if?" Happiness and forgiveness go hand-in-hand; you cannot achieve one without the other.

Lucy Hoger is a successful CEO and Senior Executive. She is a business strategist who has worked with NASDQ companies specializing in results-driven business innovation. www.lucyhoger.com.

MY REDEFINING MOMENT
SETTING A BETTER SAIL

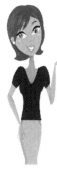

Lucy Hoger shows us that wealth is not just measured in dollars and cents, assets and acquisitions. True wealth is rooted in purpose, and produces health and happiness. How can you redefine and re-adjust your life to find your wealthy, healthy, happy place?

_____

_____

_____

_____

_____

_____

_____

PART III
REDEFINING
MOMENTS

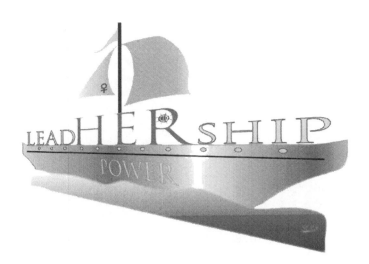

Redefining Wealth:
Quench the Thirst of Others

By Cisselon Nichols Hurd

When I was as young as three or four years old, I am told, I always had my own opinions and could articulate them well. As I grew up I loved to debate. My mother would hush me by saying, "Oh, don't make a federal case out of it." So, we got a good laugh when I was sworn in as an Assistant U.S. Attorney for the Eastern District of Texas in 1995. Mom said I had paid my dues, and now could "make a federal case out of it." How funny is that!

I've been practicing law for twenty-two years now, and am currently employed at a global integrated energy company as senior counsel, specializing in environmental law. One of my biggest legal accomplishments was working on a case that was argued before the U.S. Supreme Court. The case involved an issue of first impression under the Superfund statute and working on it was a once-in-a-life time experience.

The ultimate 8-1 ruling in our favor was huge for me personally. Most lawyers will end their careers without ever being involved in a U.S. Supreme Court case. So for me, this was gratifying!

Now I am at the top of my career and my professional journey has been fulfilling.

So is my personal life. By most people's standards and based on the taxes we pay, we are a wealthy family. I have a fantastic husband whom I adore; a lawyer himself and the son of one of the iconic Tuskegee Airmen. We have a beautiful teenage daughter and enjoy the trappings that come with a prosperous life.

Why do I tell you all this? It's my opening statement as I make my case on what true wealth really is, and what I think my real purpose is in the world.

I have been blessed and highly favored. As a result, I feel a duty to help others. My childhood circumstances and my phenomenal mother instilled in me this great sense of self pride and confidence. I have encountered a lot of people who do not have the benefit of such an upbringing. And many of them have had a lot of struggles. I am blessed with the resources to assist them, and I spend a lot of time doing just that.

Despite my challenging job that requires a lot of travel, I have always made time to support causes that I am passionate about. Once, there were so many causes my husband, who is himself very generous, had to reel me in. According to my husband, "Most people give away their money *or* their time, but not my wife; she gives away her money and her time."

Acknowledging my husband's insight caused me to become an impact giver which means I focus on certain areas and pour my time and resources into them.

One of my key focus areas is HIV/Aids. Why? A lot of people think the disease is cured since people are now able to survive if given proper medications. So society doesn't give HIV/AIDS much attention anymore. Yet, if you look at the high increase of incidents, especially among hetero-sexual African-American women, it is absolutely alarming.

My second area of focus is advancing women in the legal profession. A disturbing trend is the fact that only a small percentage of women lawyers ascend to the upper echelons of the profession. An even more disturbing trend is the high percentage of African-American female lawyers who drop out of the field entirely. This concerns me greatly, so three years ago, I became one of fifty Founders of the University of Texas Center for Women in Law (CWIL). The Center's sole purpose is to advance women in the profession.

CWIL offers a Leadership Academy which brings together law students who are in their last year of law school or first year of a judicial clerkship to be mentored and given specific tips on how to succeed in the profession. Serving as a volunteer faculty member for the Leadership Academy has given me the opportunity to share my experiences with younger women lawyers. I really enjoy this and believe that such mentoring is important. I also have mentoring relationships with lawyers who are in their twelfth year of practice, and we still have very close ties.

Another cause I champion is the military with a special focus on Wounded Warriors. I am about to ship off a bunch of Fourth of July decorations to soldiers stationed overseas so that they can have a nice Fourth of July celebration. The Sergeant who requested the decorations wants to surprise his Battalion which includes a lot of soldiers on their first deployment.

Finally and perhaps most importantly, my husband and I have a special focus on children. Through the years, we have supported many children's charities and have become personally involved helping young adults who have aged out of Foster Care.

I do believe "impact giving" is the key. You can't help everybody or solve all of the world's problems. We are only here for a short while, and there are only twenty-four hours in a day. Focusing on specific causes allows you to make a greater, more direct impact.

I probably shouldn't say out loud how much time I give to volunteerism because I don't want my husband to know. But it's upwards of twenty hours per month; probably more especially in the political season because I do a lot of voter registration and political fundraising. I'm also involved in Jack and Jill of America, Girls Inc., and several Bar Associations. And I enjoy serving on a couple of local boards.

Sure, I could just write a check. But that doesn't do it for me. I really like people and I enjoy connecting with them and if I can help them in some way, there is no greater joy.

I believe my love of giving began developing when my mother taught adult literacy after school to supplement her teacher's salary. I was in elementary school at the time and sometimes she'd take us along with her.

It was eye-opening. It was the first time I realized that there were Mommies, Daddies and Grandmas who couldn't read.

It was amazing to me when they would advance and do simple things like read their bills. I got to see a lot of their joy. So I think that experience is one of the things that really put the spark in me to help others. That joy and the ability to help is real wealth.

As a mother, a lawyer and wife I want to make sure I do everything I can to have a positive impact on the lives that I touch and society as a whole. I also want to model this behavior for my own daughter.

Why is this important? I think it's the only way to make a difference and really change the world. You have to do it person to person; one relationship, one good deed, one helping hand at a time.

My family always used to say," I'm not rich like you, girl; I can't be giving away my money." Ha! But I tell them, "Just give what you can give. Any little bit helps." All of us can help in our own way and within our individual means.

I look at people who do not help others and have no spirit of volunteerism, and I just wonder how they are fulfilled.

Generously giving my time and resources fulfills me. I don't see it as work or a chore. I am compelled to share my wealth, because my journey has been so fantastic.

I rest my case.

Cisselon Nichols Hurd is a senior counsel for a global integrated energy company specializing in environmental law.

Redefining Health:
Losing My Mind Helped Me Grow Younger

By Ellen Wood

Sometimes it's what we don't want that creates the biggest impetus for changing the course of our lives. That's what happened to me when I started following in my mother's footsteps after she wasted away with Alzheimer's.

I was in my late 50s when she died but for the previous ten years or so I had watched Mom slowly deteriorate – her mind going, then her body going. The last three plus years of her life she spent in a nursing home and every time I visited her I focused on her mental and physical decline. Mom and I had been very close but the last months of her life she didn't even know me. "Who are you?" she'd ask when I walked into her room.

I had read that Alzheimer's was hereditary so it was no surprise when I found myself in the early stages of the disease several years later. My short-term memories dissolved quickly and my tongue kept tripping on words – if I could even find the word – and I had little energy. It got so bad my kids insisted I go to the doctor for testing. Back in the late 1990's the Alzheimer's test was a series of questions the doctor would ask the patient. Well, I aced them all because I knew the answers to questions like, "What year is it?" and "Who is President of the United States?" However, because I had asked for the test it went into my medical records and when I applied for long term care insurance, they turned me down because of that test.

Then one day in 2004 I 'woke up' and realized my beliefs and programming about aging were creating a life that I did not want. I was just slipping into old age and having watched my mother, I was all too familiar with that path.

But I didn't *want* my mind and body to fall apart - I wanted to be fresh and young and alive! So right then I decided to change the course I was on. Not just to reverse my mental decline but to actually grow younger.

Once I had a clear intention to reverse aging, the next step was to learn how. I had practiced mind/spirit techniques successfully for decades to manifest my career and relationship desires – but it had never before occurred to me to use those techniques to grow younger. So I modified those mind/spirit action steps and relied on books and seminars, conferences and meditation retreats to give me additional techniques to reverse aging, including ones for the body. Soon a whole program emerged and I began making my daily youthfulness practices into habits.

My results were so astounding I had to share this information and my first book, *Think and Grow Young: Powerful Steps to Create a Life of Joy*, was born. Speaking engagements on the subject soon followed. Because this program had reversed my early stages of Alzheimer's, given me tons more energy and kept the breast cancer I had had in 1992 from recurring. I felt it was my purpose to help society change its views of what life can be in our later years. We're living longer and I had found a way to make the extended life a more dynamic and joyful experience. How could I not share it?

Today at 76 years old, I'm living proof that this program really does work. These daily practices have reversed my biological age by decades and my life is magnificent and fun. Recently on Sharon Frame's LeadHERship cruise, I donned the bright orange wig I had bought in New Orleans and strolled around the ship with a friend. You'd be amazed (I certainly was!) at the number of men, some much younger than I, who were flirting with me. And on the final evening of the cruise at the "Come As You'll Be in 2023" party, I wore a skin-tight silver sequined long dress with a side slit up to my thigh that I had bought 30 years before. It has a matching silver sequined headdress and makes me feel so glamorous. Later when I was waiting for the elevator, strangers were giving me the thumbs up and snapping my picture so I posed for them and felt like a movie star!

Act my age? I am! Inside I'm 25 and I feel fabulous. Because of my daily practices, I am more energetic, more loving, happier, wittier, my brain works better, I can dance for hours, my fingers don't hurt anymore, I look decades younger and my creativity is supercharged. Sure, I'm still a work in progress, but this is fun work! *You* can grow younger too – if you have a strong desire and are willing to take some time to do the daily practices.

But suppose you expect to just age the same way your

parents and grandparents did – what do you have to look forward to? Well, yippee! You can probably get into the movies for half price or enjoy an "early bird" dinner at a discount or have someone give up their seat for you on the bus. But along with those advantages come the aches and pains, the slow deterioration of body and mind, and the loss of memory, energy and libido.

Resolve today that that's not who you will become! Determine that you expect to have a strong, healthy body and a clear, sharp mind right up to the end. Growing younger is about being beautiful inside and out, having more joy every day that you're alive and being sexy and having fun! Two years ago I tested positive for the Alzheimer's gene, APOE-e4, but I'm still growing younger and so can you!

Ellen Wood of Taos, New Mexico is an award-winning author, speaker and columnist. Her website is www.howtogrowyounger.com. Contact her at ellen@howtogrowyounger.com.

Rejuvenate Your Life with These Practical Steps

Ellen Wood's latest book gives complete instructions for twelve daily age-reversing practices. Here they are:

- Limit sugar to twelve grams a day. Read the labels of everything for the sugar content. Cut down gradually – one day of the week at a time. Sugar causes wrinkles and depression and suppresses the immune system, among many other things detrimental to your health.
- Dry brush your skin. This not only removes dead skin cells; more importantly, it helps your lymphatic system release toxins. Get a good body brush with natural bristles – one with a long handle because you'll probably be doing this yourself (a lover might get distracted.)
- Drink half your body weight in ounces of water. Bless your water, which will make it even more beneficial.
- Observe your thoughts. The best time is when you're brushing your teeth since you don't need your conscious mind to brush your teeth – it's all muscle memory. Becoming conscious of your thoughts will change an aging mindset to a youthful outlook on life.
- Tap your way to freedom with EFT (Emotional

Freedom Technique). Negative thoughts and emotions about growing old can get stuck in your physical cellular energy system and prevent you from experiencing the joy of growing younger. Learn to release these blocks to youthfulness.

- Write an affirmation seven times. Compose a short, positive statement or use, "Every day in every way I am getting better and better." Write it four times with your dominant hand, twice with your non-dominant hand and once, more with your dominant hand. Expect to have limitless opportunities to enhance and improve your life — no matter what age you are.

- Do the Tibetan Rites of Rejuvenation. These miraculous physical movements are ancient but highly effective for growing younger. Go to my website www.howtogrowyounger.com and click on Tibetan Rites of Rejuvenation to see a video of how to perform these Rites.

- Do posture or interval training exercises. The resistance exercises for your posture are practiced in a doorway every other day. On alternate days practice quick-burst, high intensity exercises called interval training exercises.

- Exercise your brain. Yes, you can train your brain at any age! Scientific studies on neuroplasticity show that the brain is capable of creating new neuronal pathways at any age. I exercise my brain every day on www.lumosity.com but you can Google "free brain games" to avoid paying a fee.

Study, study, study. Read books that help you to be the best you can be. Go back to school or attend seminars and conferences. Keep learning.

- Choose how to respond. Learn to practice a moment of self-awareness between stimulus and response and you can clear the accumulated mental waste that manifests as symptoms of aging.

- Meditate. Regular meditation transforms you from the inside out and lets you access your deepest inner reserves for healing and living joyfully. Even five minutes a day of turning off your brain can have profound effects.

- Do something good for someone. Practice creating the world you want by calling it into being with your own generosity. Health is wealth so share the wealth. Practice daily action steps for becoming healthier and younger. Then be an example to others and show how they too can grow younger and have youthful energy and vitality and yes, even younger looks.

Redefining Happiness:
A Spring of Living Water

By The Woman at the Well

To say I have had a difficult and challenging life is a gross understatement. I've been married four times and the man I'm with now is not my husband. Life is tougher because I live in a small town where the rumor mills run constantly and everybody knows my business. I can just hear the tongues wagging as I walk through town to get to the public well. It's our only source of water, so I don't have much choice but to brave the critical looks and venture out.

My sordid record with men speaks for itself. Being "dumped" multiple times does something to your psyche, not to mention the damage to a woman's self-worth and sensibility. I believe I was happy once; at least I thought so when I flirted with men and flaunted my charm. Secret affairs came with such excitement! And indeed, "stolen water was sweeter," as the old saying goes. And "food eaten in secret did taste better." But the pleasure lasted only for a while. Then guilt would move in and overshadow me with shame.

I was itemizing my life's regrets and misery on the way to draw water at the well one day when I noticed this man standing as if he was waiting for me. "That's the last thing I needed," I said to myself, "another man to complicate my life."

As I drew nearer, I noticed something peculiar about him. First of all he didn't belong in this neighborhood. He was from a rival tribe. His people had no dealings with our kind. In fact they considered us dogs! The bad blood has existed between us for years.

So what was he doing hanging out here in public, by himself? He must have gotten lost, I thought! I noticed a kind of pleasantness about him as he asked me for a drink of water. That request alone was shocking.

And I felt compelled to speak. "Sir, why are you asking me for water? You know your people despise my people." His response ignored my question and threw me off. "If you had asked me for water," he said, "I would have given you water, but not the kind from your well."

OK, I was confused. This guy had no water bucket, and there was no other well anywhere around. So what water was he referring to?

And then he did something very strange. He started telling me about my life, reading me like a book! He revealed secrets about me only my closest friends or worst enemies would know. He brought up my long, sad history with men. But not once did he condemn me. In fact all I felt from him was love. Love from a stranger? Love from an enemy of my people? Who was this guy? He looked pretty regular, but he spoke like a prophet. So you know I had to ask. "Sir, who are you, and how do you know my tawdry secrets?

"And about this water you offer me, where is it? You have no bucket to draw water, and this well is deep."

That's when he began to tell me about the mystery he

called "living water, springing up into everlasting life." It sounded strange but somehow I felt some element of truth in his words. There was something very comforting and magnetic about this man.

His soothing voice drew me in. I didn't realize just how thirsty I was for a man to speak to me with such care. He told me if I accepted his "water" I'd never thirst again! Wow! Then it dawned on me. This living water was the very words of wisdom flowing from his lips! And I was drinking up every bit of it. This stranger assured me my checkered past could be washed away and I could start anew! You don't know how liberating those words were to a woman like me. For the first time in a long time I felt genuinely happy and hopeful.

Suddenly I started seeing myself in a better light. I was flooded with joy at just the thought of breaking free from my life of shame and regret. No, I was not a slutty, wanton woman, as some of my neighbors might have thought. Just one talk with this guy and I realized I was more than my tainted reputation. He helped me rediscover my true worth hidden under layers of wrong choices and bad behavior. He reminded me I had value! He convinced me that I mattered to God!

I was so excited I dropped my water jug and ran back home to share the news. Everybody in my town needed to hear this man's wisdom!

That day the stranger met me at the well I was broken and dejected. I thought I was beyond repair. But his loving words of wisdom began the mending process. No other man ever made me feel so very happy, so secure. I hide his words in my heart now. And yes, they are like a spring of fresh water that constantly replenishes my soul and my self-worth.

The Woman at the Well is a Bible character featured in the New Testament book of John. Read about her encounter with Jesus Christ in John 4:1-42. Note: Her portrayal in "LeadHERship" includes some editorial and imaginative reach by author, Sharon Frame.

LeadHERship's Call to Action

The woman at the well seized her LedHERship Power. She was stuck in a rut of bad choices and self-destructive behavior. But the minute she discovered she could course-correct she jumped at the chance. That's ownership; taking full responsibility for where you are in life, then making the necessary adjustments to improve.

It is not enough to be inspired by someone's encouraging words, a good book, or a soul-stirring sermon. You must pull up anchor and take action to set a better sail. Jim Rohn said, "For things to change you have to change."

LeadHERship says you've got the power to change. Take ownership of that truth and use the rudder on your vessel to steer your life. Only you can re-direct the course if you are not satisfied with your journey. Take charge!

"In the long run, we shape our lives, and we shape ourselves. The process never ends until we die. And the choices we make are ultimately our own responsibility." ~ Eleanor Roosevelt

LeadHERship says you've got the power to fix your relationships. Is an important relationship waning? Work on it. If you are not happy with the company you keep create new friendships. Loving you means not allowing toxic, life-draining people to occupy space on your ship. Toss overboard every weight that besets you. "

Never allow someone to be your priority while allowing yourself to be their option." ~ Unknown

LeadHERship says you've got the brilliance to embrace scholarship. Don't ever stop growing. Water the garden of your mind with worthy books, the arts, music, etc. Further your fascination with life itself. Be as eager as a curious child with a million and one questions. Pick up new skills, new disciplines and new hobbies. Learn all you can. Launch out into uncharted waters.

"The only person who is educated is the one who has learned how to learn and change." ~ Carl Rogers

LeadHERship says you've got what it takes to give often and generously. Never leave a person, place or thing the same way you found them. Good stewardship is the key that unlocks the door to abundance. The more you give of your time and talent, the more blessings boomerang back to you.

"The best way to find yourself is to lose yourself in the service of others." Mahatma Gandhi

LeadHERship is life itself.
Own it! Love it! Learn it! Give it!

Sharon Frame,
President of your Fan Club

ABOUT SHARON FRAME

"
Today's 'Good, Better, Best' work-shop with Sharon Frame on her LeadHERship Empowerment Cruise was amazing! Her Energy and enthusiasm will bring a new message of hope and possibility to fulfill your dream in life. "

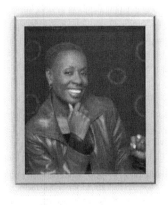

THE FORMER CNN Anchor teaches women how to "Set a better sail" in life by breaking through sabotaging blockages. Clients learn to re-frame their thinking, and retrain old habits to chart a new course in life.

Women learn to set themselves up for success by applying the four anchor principles of Ms. Frame's LeadHERship philosophy. They are: To Own. To Love. To Learn. To Give.

Ms. Frame created the LeadHERship Empowerment Cruise to give guests a relaxing, vacation get-away for leisure and learning. www.leadhershipcruise.com

Her LeadHERship Academy offers power-packed workshops and a "Focus" Mastermind group that are fun, interactive and life-transforming. www.lead-her-ship-academy.com

Ask about Ms. Frame's popular 30-Day Focus and Follow Through Challenge! It teaches clients how to turbo-charge their way to huge success by taking small, deliberate, laser-focused steps. www.focusandfollowthrough.biz

Ms. Frame is an award-winning speaker with more than 25 years of training in personal growth and self development.

Her latest book is entitled LeadHERship! Own it! Love it! Learn It! Give it: Women Redefining Wealth, Health and Happiness... And How You Can Too.

Ms. Frame's book, "Wired to Win" is powerful and practical. New York Times bestselling author Brian Tracy endorsed it. It's "The Ultimate Guide for Women Who Want to Plug In, Power Up and Push Through to Personal Greatness."

Ms. Frame has also authored "The 67th Book of the Bible: A Step-by-Step Guide to Empower You to Develop a Deeper Relationship with God, Reflect His character and to Connect to Your Greatest Potential."

LEAD**HER**ship!

Are You Ready to Launch into Your Success? Let's Go Do It!

LeadHERship Power Coach Sharon Frame offers:

▶ Focus & Follow Through 30-Day Challenge - Change your life in one month!

▶ LeadHERship Business Adjustment Bootcamp (LABB)- Secure your seat!

▶ LeadHERship "Focus" Mastermind Club- Become a high performer

▶ LeadHERship Empowerment Cruise- Come Sail with us!

▶ LeadHERship Power Party- Host one in your city!

▶ EmpowHERment Workplace Training- Invite Me

▶ EmpowHERment Speeches at conferences, big events- Book Me

▶ LeadHERship Empowerment Tour- Get on board

▶ Exclusive One-On-One Power Coaching - Invest in your success!

For details on Sharon Frame's schedule, events, book sales, special offers and bonuses, Contact Sharon Frame at www.sharonframespeaks.com or call 678-602-2899

About Our Remarkable Featured "LeadHers"

Life Re-inventor Barbara Elaine Singer is an award-winning author of *Living Without Reservations,* certified life coach and host of a week long, all-inclusive Life Reinvention Retreat in Tuscany. She has appeared on numerous TV and radio shows sharing her passion for change. Her greatest passion is to inspire others to "wake up" and start living. She specializes in overcoming fear, the power of affirmations and teaches others how to jump off the treadmill of consumerism and create a life of purpose and passion. She lives in Italy and winters in the USA. To find more information on her inspirational memoir, the retreat and life coaching practice, please go to www.HowToQuitYourLife.com

Celebrity Jewelry Designer Josette Redwolf is the quintessential jack of all trades fashion stylist, wardrobe designer to the stars. She's created jewelry and fashions for some of the biggest stars in the history of Rock n' Roll. She created her production studio in 2012 and produces "how to" videos on a wide range of the arts, as well as motivational documentaries on living with and overcoming the obstacles of chronic illness. She is a full-time wardrobe, jewelry designer and fashion stylist to celebrities and fashion photographers. Josette works along with her son Sterling to motivate and teach chronically ill and chronic pain sufferers that it's not too late to make your dreams come true. You can learn more but her work and passion at www.josetteredwolf.com; www.jredwolfproductions.com; www.josetteredwolfdesigns.com

Blind Visionary Dr. Shirley Cheng is a blind and physically disabled, award-winning author with twenty-seven book awards. She is a Bible teacher and proclaimer of the good news of salvation through Jesus Christ. Dr. Cheng is founder of www.Ultra-Ability.com Ministry, summa cum laude graduate with Doctor of Divinity, motivational speaker, poet, and author of nine books. She has also contributed to over twenty-five other books. Shirley has had severe juvenile rheumatoid arthritis since infancy. Owing to years of hospitalization, she received no education until age eleven. Back then, she knew only her ABCs and very simple English. However, after only about 180 days of special education in elementary school, she mastered grade level and entered a regular sixth grade class in middle school. Unfortunately, Shirley lost her eyesight at the age of seventeen. After successful eye surgery, she hopes to earn multiple science doctorates from Harvard University. You can find out more about Shirley's free Bible study classes at www.ShirleyCheng.com

Homeless to Millionaire! Shanna McFarlane is known as the Power-house Entrepreneur who went from "Homeless on the Streets to Owning the Street!" She is a recognized leader and the new voice for personal and entrepreneurial success! Shanna went from a life of many challenges and adversities including being homeless at the tender age of 16; against the odds she changed the outcome of her life by changing the script chapter by chapter – going on to build a multi-million dollar real estate business and founded several other profitable and successful businesses, some of which she started from the trunk of her car! Shanna was named a nominee for the prestigious *RBC 2012 & 2013 Canadian Woman Entrepreneur of the Year Award* and is recognized as one of Canada's most powerful women in real estate investing. Her life has served as one of influence, one that inspires hope, empowers success & transforms the lives of thousands of men and women around the globe to work toward achieving a life of personal & entrepreneurial success! www.shannamcfarlane.com

Business Strategist: Lucy Hoger is a successful CEO and Senior Executive with a track record for propelling organizations and companies to the next level of profitable achievement within highly competitive markets. She has proven herself repeatedly as a leader for spearheading the turnaround of potential business failures into successes. She possess an exceptional ability to develop and retain leadership teams comprised of the "best of the best" talent that creates results-driven technology and business innovation. Her unique expertise was honed through her background as a strategic consultant with Price Waterhouse and Gemini Consulting. That experience, combined with her background in real-world performance for several NASDQ companies, brings a unique insight into problem solving for any business situation. www.lucyboger.com.

Impact Giver: Cisselon Nichols Hurd is a mother, wife and lawyer. She serves as senior counsel for a global integrated energy company specializing in environmental law. She has also served in a variety of governmental positions in the U.S. Virgin Islands, including Counsel to the Attorney General and Assistant Attorney General for Environmental Enforcement. Ms. Hurd also worked at the U.S. Department of Justice in the Attorney General's Honors Program as a Trial Attorney in the Environment and Natural Resources Division and as an

Assistant United States Attorney in the Eastern District of Texas where she prosecuted environmental crimes. Ms. Hurd obtained her B.A. and B.S. degree from the University of Texas at Austin. She also received her law degree from the University of Texas.

Grow Young Guide Ellen Wood is an award-winning author, columnist and speaker. As a carrier of the Alzheimer's gene, APOE-e4, Ellen is proving she can keep that gene in the 'off' position with practices that strengthen and invigorate mind, body and spirit. She offers herself as living proof that these practices work. Her latest book, *Rejuvenate Your Life*, is the powerful step-by-step program that combines cutting-edge research in neuroscience and cell biology with ancient esoteric teachings and a deep trust in Spirit and the power of the mind. This practical self-help approach of 12 daily practices is interspersed with engaging, amusing anecdotes of how the author encountered, challenged and overcame old paradigms about aging.
www.HotToGrowYounger.com

57016972R00075

Made in the USA
Lexington, KY
06 November 2016